Praise for Bryan Doerries's

THE THEATER OF WAR

"The theater of ancient Greece was many things. . . . [It is] the therapeutic potential of catharsis that most interests Bryan Doerries. . . . An impressive and accomplished journey."
—James Shapiro,
The New York Times Book Review

"Extraordinary. . . . Riveting. . . . [Doerries] discussed *Ajax* with many troubled vets returning from Iraq and Afghanistan, and may have saved some of their lives. His book interweaves tales from this journey with episodes from Doerries's own life and moving discussions of the plays he cherishes—his 'blueprints for felt experience,' his conduits for connection and compassion. . . . It is through that intensity of focus, Doerries convinces us, that we can find permission to feel our own pain. To see his productions today, or to see Greek tragedy through his eyes, is to become measurably healthier and more human."
—James Romm, *The Daily Beast*

"The route Bryan Doerries describes in his memoir is as unique as the place it landed him. . . . Moving. . . . Doerries's book loops around from autobiography to literary analysis to medical ethics and back again. . . . It should win him a host of new admirers."
—*The New York Times*

"Doerries's account of his performances with Theater of War is at once an impassioned history lesson, a manual of therapy for the afflicted and a deep analysis of the power of ancient Greek tragedy."

—*The Wichita Eagle*

"Important and illuminating. . . . This is an admirable book about an admirable project."

—Andrew J. Bacevich, *The American Scholar*

"Bryan Doerries has given us a gift to be treasured."

—Tim O'Brien

"In this riveting narrative, simply but elegantly told, Doerries movingly resurrects the inner life of a people who lived twenty-five hundred years ago, but whose struggles evoke our own familiar and damaged present, now endowed by this wonderful book with more drama, more tragedy, more compassion, more possibility. Here is the proof at last: our future depends on the gifts of the past."

—Ken Burns

"A testament both to the enduring power of the classics and to the vital role art can play in our communal understanding of war and suffering."

—Phil Klay, author of *Redeployment*

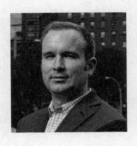

Bryan Doerries

THE THEATER OF WAR

Bryan Doerries is a writer, director, and translator. He is the founder of Theater of War, a project that presents readings of ancient Greek plays to service members, veterans, and their families to help them initiate conversations about the visible and invisible wounds of war. He is also the cofounder of Outside the Wire, a social-impact company that uses theater and a variety of other media to address pressing public health and social issues, such as combat-related psychological injury, end-of-life care, prison reform, domestic violence, political violence, recovery from natural and man-made disasters, and addiction. A self-described "evangelist" for classical literature and its relevance to our lives today, Doerries uses age-old approaches to help individuals and communities heal after suffering and loss.

www.outsidethewirellc.com

ALSO BY BRYAN DOERRIES

All That You've Seen Here Is God:
New Versions of Four Greek Tragedies:
Sophocles' Ajax, Philoctetes, *and* Women of Trachis
& Aeschylus' Prometheus Bound

The Odyssey of Sergeant Jack Brennan

THE
THEATER
OF
WAR

THE
THEATER
OF
WAR

What Ancient Greek Tragedies
Can Teach Us Today

Bryan Doerries

VINTAGE BOOKS
A Division of Penguin Random House LLC
New York

FIRST VINTAGE BOOKS EDITION, AUGUST 2016

Copyright © 2015 by Bryan Doerries

All rights reserved. Published in the United States by Vintage Books, a division of Penguin Random House LLC, New York, and distributed in Canada by Random House of Canada, a division of Penguin Random House Canada Limited, Toronto. Originally published in hardcover in the United States by Alfred A. Knopf, a division of Penguin Random House LLC, New York, in 2015.

Vintage and colophon are registered trademarks of Penguin Random House LLC.

Grateful acknowledgment is made to *The Falmouth Enterprise* for permission to reprint three separate Letters to the Editor (July 15, 2011). Reprinted by permission of *The Falmouth Enterprise*.

The Library of Congress has cataloged the Knopf edition as follows:
Doerries, Bryan, author.
The theater of war: what ancient Greek tragedies can teach us today / Bryan Doerries.
pages cm
Includes bibliographical references.
1. Greek drama (Tragedy)—History and criticism.
2. War in literature.   I. Title.
PA3136.D65 2015   882'.0109—dc23   2014049746

Vintage Books Trade Paperback ISBN: 978-0-307-94972-1
eBook ISBN: 978-0-307-95946-1

Author photograph © Howard Korn
Book design by Betty Lew

www.vintagebooks.com

Printed in the United States of America
10 9 8 7 6 5 4 3 2

For my wife, Sarah, and our daughter, Abigail

People have always endeavored to understand antiquity by means of the present—and shall the present now be understood by means of antiquity?

—FRIEDRICH NIETZSCHE,
We Philologists

CONTENTS

THE
THEATER
OF
WAR

PROLOGUE

Standing before a crowd of war-weary infantry soldiers after a reading of Sophocles's *Ajax* on a U.S. Army installation in southwestern Germany, I posed the following question, one that I have asked tens of thousands of service members and veterans on military bases all over the world: "Why do you think Sophocles wrote this play?"

Ajax tells the story of a formidable Greek warrior who loses his friend Achilles in the ninth year of the Trojan War, falls into a depression, is passed over for the honor of inheriting Achilles's armor, and attempts to kill his commanding officers. Feeling betrayed and overcome with blind rage, Ajax slaughters a herd of cattle, mistaking them for his so-called enemies. When he finally realizes what he has done—covered in blood and consumed with shame—he takes his own life by hurling his body upon a sword.

The play was written nearly twenty-five hundred years ago by a Greek general and was performed in the center of Athens for thousands of citizen-soldiers during a century in which the Athenians saw nearly eighty years of war. And yet the story is as contemporary as this morning's news. According to a 2012 Veterans Affairs study, an average of twenty-two U.S. veterans take their own lives each day. That's almost one suicide per hour.

A junior enlisted soldier, seated in the third row, raised his hand and matter-of-factly replied, "He wrote it to boost morale."

I stepped closer to him and asked, "What is morale-boosting about watching a decorated warrior descend into madness and take his own life?"

"It's the truth," he replied—subsumed in a sea of green uniforms—"and we're all here watching it together."

The soldier had highlighted something hidden within *Ajax:* a message for our time. Sophocles didn't whitewash the horrors of war. This wasn't government-sponsored propaganda. Nor was his play an act of protest. It was the unvarnished truth. And by presenting the truth of war to combat veterans, he sought to give voice to their secret struggles and to convey to them that they were not alone.

On March 20, 2003, I lost my twenty-two-year-old girlfriend, Laura Rothenberg, to cystic fibrosis. Twenty months earlier she had received a double lung transplant, and although she survived the procedure, no surgery or drug could ultimately halt the slow, steady decline, as her immune system rejected the new organs. As she approached death, her fear of dying seemed to intensify. Breathing itself became an ordeal, as her inflamed lungs scraped against the inside of her chest with every breath.

On the last day of her life, six weeks after her twenty-second birthday, Laura called her family and closest friends to her bedside, unstrapped her oxygen mask, and proceeded to comfort those of us around her with assuring words. Then, quietly, gracefully, she stopped breathing and died.

Laura was the last of more than twenty of her childhood friends to succumb to cystic fibrosis, a genetic disorder that afflicts nearly thirty thousand people—mostly children—every year. The friends she had grown up with had become like siblings, over long hospital stays at Columbia-Presbyterian, and all had predeceased her. She often asked me why she alone had survived. My answer was always the same: to tell the story.

Three months after Laura's death, her memoir—*Breathing for a Living*—was released. The book chronicles her experience undergoing a double lung transplant and the impact of the surgery on those around her. While she was not well enough to write about the final chapter of her life, she was able to dictate an epilogue to me. The last line of the book poses a seemingly unanswerable question: "How can I resign myself to death if I am still afraid of not being able to breathe?" It was a question that had consumed her for nearly twenty-two years, and which she definitively answered in the final moments of her life.

For weeks after her death, all I wanted to do was talk about it to anyone who would listen. But after her memorial, fewer and fewer people wanted to hear the story. Nevertheless, I kept telling it—in all its graphic detail—even as people seemed to recoil from the manic intensity of my monologue. I needed friends and family members, and even strangers, to know that her death was brave and poetic and transcendent and beautiful, and that it was possible for someone to die fully conscious and connected with those she loved.

In the following years, whenever I returned to the ancient Greek tragedies I had studied in college, the conflicted, suffering characters in the plays spoke to me with an immediacy that I never could have anticipated before caring for Laura. I took comfort in knowing that I wasn't the first person who had experienced compassion fatigue, or who had hesitated to act decisively in the presence of extreme suffering, or who felt ambivalent about helping someone to die, or whose grief manifested itself in a withdrawal from the world. If ancient Greek tragedies could speak directly to me, I reasoned, they could also speak to anyone who had lived the human experiences they described. And if there's one thing I've since learned from listening to audiences all over the world respond to Greek tragedy, it's that people who have come into contact with death, who have faced the darkest aspects of our humanity, who have loved and lost, and who know the meaning of sacrifice, seem to have little trouble relating to these ancient plays. These tragedies are their stories.

What do Greek tragedies have to say to us now? What timeless things do they show us about what it means to be human? What were these ancient plays originally designed to do? And can they still work for audiences and readers today? These are some of the questions that I have been exploring with unconventional audiences in unlikely settings. Over the past decade, I have directed readings of my translations of Greek tragedies and other ancient texts for thousands of combat veterans, hospice nurses, cancer patients, recovering addicts, homeless men and women, doctors, social workers, disaster victims, and corrections officers, all over the world. I've directed performances in far-flung places, such as Germany, Scandinavia, Japan, Kuwait, Qatar, and even Guantánamo Bay, Cuba; and I've also directed them at venues closer to home, such as the Brooklyn Academy of Music (less than a block from where I live with my wife and daughter).

In the beginning, I went searching for audiences that, by virtue of their life experiences, would respond directly and powerfully to these ancient plays, but in recent years new audiences have begun seeking me out— and my theater company, Outside the Wire—to ask, "Do you know of a play that could help our community deal with what we've been through?" Each performance has led to the next, and each community has opened doors to others, expanding the reach of the work, like an infinite series of concentric circles all rippling out from the same point of impact.

I am a self-proclaimed evangelist for classical literature and its relevance to our lives today. It is my belief that ancient Greek tragedies have something urgent to show us about ourselves, something that we desperately need to see. The goal of this book is not to make easy connections between the ancient past and the present, but to listen closely to ancient tragedies and ask, "What do we recognize of ourselves and our struggles in these stories?" This is a book about how and why Greek tragedies can help us face some of the most complex issues of our time, shedding light on universal human experiences, illuminating the moral and spiritual dimensions of trauma and loss.

I am not a professor, and this is not a work of scholarship. All the translations of Greek tragedies within these pages are mine. However, they are not literal word-for-word renderings of Greek into English, but rather adaptive attempts to convey the drive and action of Greek drama, clearly and directly, for contemporary readers. This is not a traditional book about why we should read the classics. It is about the power of tragedies to transcend time, to comfort the afflicted and afflict the comfortable. At its core, it is about how stories can help us heal and possibly even change, before it's too late.

LEARNING THROUGH SUFFERING

I

In the fall of fourth grade, I landed a small role in a production of Euripides's *Medea* at the local community college in Newport News, Virginia, where my father taught experimental psychology. I played one of the ill-fated boys slaughtered at the hand of their pathologically jealous mother. I can still remember my one line, which I belted backstage with abandon as several drama majors pretended to bludgeon me with long wooden canes behind a black velvet curtain—"No, no, the sword is falling!" The director, a short, fiery German auteur with spiky white hair and a black leather jacket always draped over his shoulders like a cape, would scream at the cast during rehearsals at the top of his lungs until we delivered our lines with the appropriate zeal. Whenever our performances reached the desired fever pitch, he would jump up from his chair and explode with delight, "Now veeee are koooooking!"

During daytime performances for local high school students, the boredom in the theater was as palpable as the thick layer of humidity generated by sweaty adolescents fidgeting in their seats, whispering and blowing spitballs in the shadows, waiting for the agony to end. Whenever I entered the stage, wearing a tight gold polyester tunic, which clung to my thighs and itched mercilessly under the unforgiving lights, I heard rippling waves of laughter move through the crowd. *What's so funny?* I wondered, squinting into the stage lights. After the show closed, at the cast party, one of my fellow actors confirmed that the laughter had, in fact, been at my expense. Unaccustomed to wearing a tunic, I had provided the high school audiences with an extended, full frontal view of my underwear while perched atop a large granite boulder. Seeing my Fruit of the Looms was likely the most memorable event in those students' mandatory encounter with Euripides.

Most of us probably developed an allergy to ancient Greek drama in high school, when some well-intending English teacher required us to read plays like *Oedipus the King, Antigone, Prometheus Bound,* and *The Oresteia* in rigid Victorian translation, or forced us to watch seemingly endless films featuring British actors in loose-fitting sheets and golden sandals declaiming the vocative refrain "O, Zeus!" from behind masks. If your early encounters with the ancient Greeks zapped you of any ambition to ever pick up a play by Aeschylus, Sophocles, or Euripides again, you are not alone. Aeschylus is known for having written in his play *Agamemnon* that humans "learn through suffering," but for most students, studying ancient Greek drama is just an exercise in suffering, with no apparent educational value.

Ironically, some scholars now suggest that attending the dramatic festivals in ancient Greece and watching plays by the great tragic poets served as an important rite of passage for late-adolescent males, known as *ephebes.* It is for this reason, according to the argument, that so many of the tragedies feature teenage characters—such as Antigone, Pentheus, Neoptolemus, and Orestes—thrust into ethically fraught situations with no easy answers and in which someone is likely to die. According to this understanding, tragedy may have been viewed as formalized training, preparing late adolescents for the ethical and emotional challenges of adult life, including military service and civic participation. In other words, the very plays that were designed thousands of years ago to educate and engage teenagers, to help transform them from children into productive citizens, have managed to bore them senseless for centuries.

One hope of this book is to administer an antidote to the obligatory high school unit on ancient Greek tragedy.

The first thing you learn in school about tragedy is that it tells the story of a good and prosperous individual who is brought to ruin by some defect in his or her character. This traditional reading of Greek tragedy goes something like this: Blinded by pride, or *hubris,* Oedipus ignores the warning of an oracle, unwittingly murders his father and sleeps with his mother, and— though he manages to save the people of Thebes from the bloodthirsty Sphinx—ultimately turns out to be the contagion that is plaguing his city. Conclusion: Oedipus was a great but flawed individual who was deluded by power and crushed by external forces beyond his grasp. We love stories about well-intentioned, flawed characters, because they make the most compelling drama. Also, as Aristotle pointed out, we take no pleasure in watching morally flawless people suffer.

But the ancient Greek word commonly translated in textbooks as "flaw," *hamartia,* more accurately means "error," from the verb *hamartano,* "to miss the mark." Centuries later, by the time of the New Testament, the same word—*hamartia*—came to mean "sin," fully loaded with all its moral judgment. In other words, tragedies depict characters making mistakes, rather than inherent flaws in character. I know that I miss the mark hundreds of times each day. I often have to lose my way in order to find the right path forward. Making mistakes, even habitually and unknowingly, is central to what it means to be human. Characters in Greek tragedies stray, err, and get lost. They are no more flawed than the rest of humanity; the difference lies in the scale of their mistakes, which inevitably cost lives and ruin generations.

At the same time, being human and making mistakes—even in ignorance—does not absolve these tragic characters of responsibility for their actions. Had they fully understood what they were doing, they most certainly wouldn't have done it. But they did it all the same. It is in this gray zone—at the thin border between

ignorance and responsibility—that ancient Greek tragedies play out. This is one of the many reasons that tragedies still speak to us with undiminished force today. We
all live in that gray zone, in which we are neither condemned by nor absolved of our mistakes.

What is so utterly flawed about the idea of the "tragic
flaw" is that it encourages us to judge rather than to
empathize with characters like Oedipus. Tragedies are
designed not to teach us morals but rather to validate
our moral distress at living in a universe in which many
of our actions and choices are influenced by external
powers far beyond our comprehension—such as luck,
fate, chance, governments, families, politics, and genet-
ics. In this universe, we are dimly aware, at best, of the
sum total of our habits and mistakes, until we have
unwittingly destroyed those we love or brought about
our own destruction.

It is not our job to judge the characters in Greek
tragedies—to focus on their "flaws." Tragedy challenges us to see ourselves in the way its characters stray
from the path, and to open our eyes to the bad habits
we may have formed or to the mistakes we have yet to
make. Contrary to what you may have learned in school,
tragedies are not designed to fill us with pessimism and
dread about the futility of human existence or our relative powerlessness in a world beyond our grasp. They
are designed to help us see the impending disaster on
the horizon, so that we may correct course and nar-
rowly avoid it. Above all, the flaw in our thinking about
tragedy is that we look for meaning where there is none

to be found. Tragedies don't *mean* anything. They *do* something.

Another concept that gets drilled into our heads in high school is "fate." The word for *fate* in ancient Greek—*moira*—means "portion." In Greek antiquity, Fate was worshipped in the form of three goddesses: Clotho, the "spinner"; Lachesis, the "allotter"; and Atropos, the "unturnable." Fate was older and more powerful than all the gods combined, and the entire cosmos was subject to its laws. No one lived above it or beyond it. Yet the Greek concept of fate, as it is encountered in Greek tragedy, is much subtler than many of us generally understand. In tragedy, the concept of fate is not mutually exclusive of the existence of free will; nor does the ancient idea of "destiny" negate the role of personal choice and human agency. In fact, as in the case of Oedipus, human choices and actions are required in order to fulfill an individual's fate or destiny.

In 1976, the year I was born, my father was diagnosed with type 2 diabetes, an insidious, cruel disease that dismantled his mind and body slowly, almost imperceptibly, over a period of thirty-three years. In spite of the diagnosis, he adamantly refused to adjust his lifestyle, though he knew this choice would eventually come at a deadly cost. The nerves in his feet died first. Then the bones in his ankles collapsed. Then came the incurable lesions, the festering sores, the bouts of colitis, the kidney failure, the daily dialysis treatments, the kidney transplant, the septic infections, the endocarditis, the blindness, the dementia, the seizures, the horrifying hallucinations, and finally—after much suffering—a protracted, terrifying death, during the final days of which he believed a gaggle of black, ravenlike demons were swarming all around him, waiting to take his soul to hell.

The word *diabetes* comes from the Greek verb *diabaino,* "to run through." The name derives from the signature symptoms of the disease, an unquenchable thirst combined with a constant need to urinate. Water "runs through" diabetics. The condition results from a deficiency in the pancreas, which normally produces insulin, a hormone that regulates sugar levels in the blood. Without enough insulin, sugars run wild, causing, among other symptoms, extreme thirst while steadily choking off the blood supply to nerves and tissues. Ultimately, over decades, the disease leaves no organ unscathed.

Type 2 diabetes is a fitting metaphor for the human condition as portrayed in ancient Greek tragedy, and for the interdependence of human action and fate. Those who are diagnosed with the disease often possess a genetic predisposition to develop it. It is written into their DNA, like an ancient intergenerational curse. And yet what diabetics choose to do with the knowledge of their condition has a direct impact upon their lives, and upon those who love them. Thus, in spite of the "curse" of their disease, diabetics still play a role in shaping their destiny. How they behave and the choices they make help determine the course their lives will take. Many are able to control their blood sugars through a combination of drugs, diet, and exercise, extending their life spans and delaying the progression of the disease for decades. But as many as 60 percent of type 2 diabetics do not adhere to the recommendations of their doctors or faithfully take their medication. This is primarily because diabetics do not experience for years the negative effects of eating junk food, not exercising, and allowing blood sugars to fluctuate. It is also because the medical regimen for most full-blown diabetics involves daily injections of insulin and constant monitoring of sugars with needle pricks to well-worn fingertips.

Fate refers to the cards we were dealt, the *portion* we were given at birth. Tragedy depicts how our choices and actions shape our destiny. No one ever said that change was easy, but my father believed it was impossible. He often told his experimental psychology students that when it comes to human behavior, what passes for change is no more than a fantasy, an illusion. This was his long-formed, heavily entrenched conviction, based on years of research, working with human beings and rats.

Nothing infuriated me more than to listen to him rationalize his own self-destruction with this specious argument. His unwillingness to acknowledge even the remote possibility of meaningful change fueled some of our worst fights and forever drove a wedge between us.

In the heat of one memorable argument, he eyed the collection of Sophocles's plays I had under my arm and asked, "Don't you believe in fate, Bryan? All those

Greek plays end in disaster, no matter what the characters try to do."

Like Oedipus, my father was adopted, but he wasn't told until much later, so he spent the entirety of his childhood believing that his adoptive parents were his biological parents. And like Oedipus, he discovered who his biological parents were near the end of his life, when it was too late to act upon this knowledge and avert his own self-destruction. In Sophocles's version of the Oedipus myth, a Corinthian man, in a moment of inebriated indiscretion, accuses Oedipus of being a bastard, planting the seed that, decades later, bears fruit in the horrifying realization of his true identity. When my father turned sixteen, it was his grandmother, Hattie, who took him aside and casually, one might say cruelly, shattered his world by telling him he was adopted.

Decades later, while searching for a viable kidney donor for my father, we found out who his biological parents were. As fate would have it, they both worked at the Catholic hospital in Fairhaven, New Jersey, where he had been born. My father's father had been his pediatrician, a Spanish immigrant, who had indulged in an extramarital affair with a Puerto Rican nurse. My father's adoptive parents, who were in their forties and had been unable to conceive, were more than willing to help the physician and the nurse sweep their dalliance under the rug by taking the baby off their hands. Had it not been for my great-grandmother's loose lips, they might have perpetuated the myth that he was their son for the rest of their lives.

According to the Centers for Disease Control and Prevention, Hispanic Americans are at a "particularly high risk for type 2 diabetes." My father's fate, as it turned out, was something he could have, at the very least, deferred, had he investigated the identity of his biological parents. But like Oedipus, he did not really want to know the truth until it was too late. When Oedipus discovers who his parents were, he gouges out his eyes with golden pins from his mother's gown and stumbles off into the desert to die. My father drank a chocolate milk shake and slipped off into sugar-induced oblivion.

A week before my father died, frail and demented, at the age of sixty-six, I flew down from New York City to visit him at a nursing home in Virginia, a few blocks from where I had grown up. I brought him a chocolate milk shake from Monty's Penguin, the local diner we had frequented during my childhood. Though neither of us wanted to say goodbye, we both knew it was the last time we would see each other. After a long day of reminiscing and grappling with unanswerable questions, we eventually ran out of things to say.

The sun had already set, though I hadn't noticed its absence until after the room faded to black and the floodlights outside poured through cracks in the blinds, crisscrossing the floor. We sat in the darkness for an indeterminate time and looked at each other with understanding and regret. Finally, after my father closed his eyes and slipped back into semiconsciousness, I tossed my coat over my shoulder and slowly approached his bed, bending over to look at him one last time, to take in his face, so I wouldn't somehow forget its contours after he was gone.

Suddenly, without opening his eyes, he reached up and grabbed my arm, pulling me toward his face—contorted in a rictus of horror—with the desperation of a drowning victim. Clamping down with all his remaining strength, he sobbed: "The same thing is going to happen to you, and to your brother! It's fate. It's fate!"

It's his dementia talking, I told myself, *not him.* But it was also a curse.

As a child, I often spent afternoons observing him train his advanced psychology students in a small laboratory a few blocks from our house. Among the many wonders of that mysterious windowless space was a floor-to-ceiling polygraph machine, a shriveled human brain floating in a glass jar of formaldehyde, and rows of metal cages packed with albino lab rats, peeking between bars with beady red eyes. In one experiment, which I observed at perhaps too young an age to fully understand, he demonstrated how rats would eventually give up their will to live if provided enough negative reinforcement, through a series of seemingly indiscriminate electrical shocks. Eventually, when they'd had enough, the rats stopped struggling, rested their heads on the floors of their cages, opened their mouths, and simply waited to die.

Now, as I left the nursing home and rushed to my

car, with my father's last words still echoing in my ears, it occurred to me that the curse of his interpretation of fate was that it permitted him to act like those rats. Did he somehow expect me to do the same? Was this the lesson he wanted me to learn from tragedy?

For my father, fate was a pretext to behave fatalistically. It was the same notion of "inescapable fate" that I had encountered in school. Whenever I heard it, every cell in my body rose up in revolt, resisting the idea that we humans live without the ability to change the course of our destinies. Thinking about the way my father placed the concept of fate at the center of his self-destructive, pessimistic worldview, I couldn't help believing that the objective of ancient Greek tragedy—and its grim depiction of humanity—was radically different from what we have imagined for thousands of years.

Fate and free will are not mutually exclusive in ancient Greek tragedy. Fate always requires human action—or inaction—in order to be fulfilled. Perhaps by cultivating a heightened awareness of the forces that shape our lives and of the pivotal role our choices and actions play in realizing our destiny, Greek tragedy was designed to promote the possibility of change. In other words, the fate that awaited Oedipus was avoidable, as was my father's. So is yours, and so is mine.

II

Although I first encountered Greek tragedy in elementary school, it wasn't until my first year at Kenyon, a small liberal arts college in rural Ohio with a rich literary history, that I became interested in the classical world, for all the wrong reasons.

The classicist and philosopher Friedrich Nietzsche once wrote:

1. A young man cannot have the slightest conception of what the Greeks and Romans were.
2. He doesn't know whether he is fitted to investigate them.

In his 1874 essay *We Philologists,* a wry polemic against nineteenth-century German classicism, Nietzsche argues that young students are poorly suited to study the ancients precisely because they lack the life experience to understand the motivations and struggles of other humans, let alone those who lived more than two thousand years before them. Even worse off than students in this regard, suggests Nietzsche, are career academics.

"The philologist," he writes, "must first of all be a man." *Philologist* in Greek means "lover of words," and for centuries the term has denoted the profession of studying ancient languages and cultures. Nietzsche argues, tongue firmly planted in his cheek, "Old men are well suited to be philologists if they were not such during the portion of their lives which was richest in experiences." In other words, only those who have lived the extremities of life—who have loved, traveled, risked, lost, and suffered—can extract anything of value from reading the ancients. Conversely, he suggests, studying philology can get in the way of living a full, rich life. "In short," he concludes, with a playful jab at his critics, "ninety-nine philologists out of a hundred should not be philologists at all." At the core of Nietzsche's argument lies the concept that experience is a prerequisite for understanding the ancient world.

At age eighteen, with relatively little life experience, I signed up for two semesters of ancient Greek, in a class that met for several hours a day, Monday through Friday, and set out to prove to myself that I had what it took to investigate the Greeks. The four other students in my class and I convened daily around a large, stately oak table on the first floor of a neo-Gothic building, complete with gargoyles and soaring stained-glass windows. On the first day of class, the legendary professor Bill McCulloh, a former Rhodes scholar from Ohio and then chair of the classics department, passed around a short survey that included the question "Why are you interested in studying ancient Greek?"

My response, in retrospect, was embarrassingly naïve: "In pursuit of esoteric knowledge." I somehow envisioned ancient Greek to be an initiation, a rigorous course of study that would provide access to a hidden world, such as the Eleusinian Mysteries, famously secret rites and ceremonies held each year in honor of the goddesses Demeter and Persephone. Nietzsche was right. I hadn't the slightest clue as to who the Greeks and Romans were. But I possessed a burning desire to find out.

In his *Poetics,* an unfinished collection of lecture notes on Greek tragedy and other forms of poetry written during the fourth century BC, Aristotle defines tragedy as the *mimesis* of *praxis,* or the "representation of an action." According to the philosopher, tragedy was a highly technical form of storytelling, in which—above all other elements—plot mattered most.

People don't tend to think of tragedy in this way. They associate it with synchronized gestures and over-wrought displays of emotions rather than with tightly woven storylines that move with the precision of Swiss clocks. However, Aristotle argues that the logical progression of a well-constructed story, in which events flow in natural succession, brings human behaviors to life. "Tragedy," he writes, "is a representation not of people as such but of actions and life." It is through unfolding dramatic action that characters are portrayed. Without action—that is, characters making "moral choices"—there is no character, only *characterization.* In other words, in tragedies, characters are defined by what they do, not by what they say or what is said about them. The ancient Greek word *kharakter,* or "type, nature, character," comes from a verb that means "to engrave." Drawing upon this metaphor, the pre-Socratic philosopher Heraclitus is known to have said, "A person's character is his fate." In other words, our destiny is etched or engraved upon us by our thoughts and choices.

The word *drama* comes from the Greek verb *drao,*

"to act or do." Many scholars trace the origins of tragedy back to the first known actor, Thespis, a sixth-century BC singer of dithyrambs, choral odes about well-known mythological subjects. Thespis did something remarkable when he first took on the personae of individual characters, telling stories from their perspectives, enacting behavior. Though the story of Thespis is likely no more than a myth, constructed to explain how tragedy evolved from other poetic forms, the impulse during the sixth century BC to *enact*, rather than simply recount, stories was central to the development of tragedy.

What sets Greek tragedies apart from many other texts that have survived from the ancient world is that they were written for performance. These plays don't live on the page. They demand to be enacted or staged, and though Aristotle claimed that reading them achieved the same effect as seeing them, I believe we must experience them in order to understand them, because tragedy is less a literary form than a blueprint for a felt experience. Performed live, in the presence of an audience, tragedy accomplishes what it was designed to do.

For centuries, Greek tragedies have been viewed as cultural or aesthetic artifacts of the ancient world that impart age-old adages about the human condition to passive audiences. But we must invert the equation. It is by actively recognizing our behaviors and actions in these ancient stories that we imbue them with significance. Tragedies embody basic human behavior in order that we might see it as our own.

Learning ancient Greek at Kenyon College proved grueling, and by the end of that first semester, my desk and my life had been overtaken by flash cards, lexicons, spiral notebooks brimming with morphologies, and critical commentaries. While I wasn't a quick student—I've never been especially adept at learning languages—I was the most dedicated student in the class. On many mornings I would be the first person to enter the dining hall, the first to trudge down the long gravel path that led through the center of campus, and the first to flip on the lights in the dark-paneled classroom where I would chant declensions over strong black coffee until the other students arrived, two hours later, to begin the daily drudgery of quizzes and drills.

Halfway through the second semester, after slogging through sections of Plato's *Crito* and wondering, bleary-eyed, whether I had the resolve to someday make it through Homer's *Odyssey* or Thucydides's *History of the Peloponnesian War,* we started reading sections of Euripides's *Medea.*

One night while translating an especially difficult passage, I slammed the text shut in frustration and put my head in my hands. I began to imagine how I might stage the final scene of the play, in which the aggrieved sorceress Medea murders her two young boys in order to punish her unfaithful husband, Jason. In the final moments of the play, she appears with their corpses in a magical chariot flying high above the stage. I distantly remembered the scene from the community college production of my childhood, and I soon found myself swept up in the story. Like the fiery German director of that production, I began goading imaginary actors as the tragedy played out in my mind, until they delivered their lines with the intensity of first responders pulling small corpses from the rubble of a collapsed building.

Then it was dawn.

In ancient Greek from the classical period, there are two words for time—*chronos,* or chronological, everyday time, and *kairos,* the right moment, the moment that should be seized, or that seizes you. I can count on my fingers the number of instances I have experienced a true *kairos,* a moment in which the impulse to act is coupled by an immediate, intuitive understanding of precisely what to do. In each instance, the experience has heralded something life-changing on the horizon. And so it was while reading Euripides's *Medea* in ancient Greek, ten years after playing one of her unlucky children, that I first sensed what I would one day do with my burgeoning classical education and felt the pull of what could only be described as a calling.

What was the role of myth in the ancient world, and what can myths do for us today? The Romanian scholar of comparative religion Mircea Eliade popularized a concept in the early 1950s called the "eternal return," which, however dated, still goes a long way toward answering these questions. Eliade spent his life studying the spiritual behavior of tribal cultures in remote parts of the world that were still practicing the atavistic rituals and religions of their ancient ancestors. Based on what he found, he argued that human beings are universally and cross-culturally hardwired to respond to rituals and myths. Through the retelling of myths, archaic humans imbued their otherwise unremarkable lives with significance. Today myths disrupt the everyday experience of time by transporting us back to the beginning.

Before recorded history, human experience was interpreted, contextualized, and understood through myths about the origins of the cosmos and its inhabitants. In other words, the ancient experience of reality was mediated by mythology. For archaic humans, states Eliade, "an object or an act becomes real only insofar as it imitates or repeats an archetype," or an original act. Marriage was significant in relation to the original marriage of the first man and woman, or the marriage of the gods. The passage from adolescence into adulthood was significant in relation to the coming of age of the first man. According to Eliade, through the ritualized reenactment of myths, in ceremonies and rites, the lives of archaic humans were merged with the archetypal stories of heroes, ancestors, and gods. Myth was, and still is, a vehicle for bringing our lives into contact with something deep within us and larger than ourselves.

While much of the secular, industrialized world has lost touch with the power of rituals and myth, humans today are no less receptive to them than were our ancient forebears. We still ache for contact with the transcendent and the divine. We yearn to know that we are part of something bigger. And we are relieved to discover that we are not alone, especially across time.

The word *sophomore* comes from two Greek roots: *sophos,* "wise"; and *moros,* "foolish." During my sophomore year of college, in an act of blind ambition, I determined to take on the entire classical tripod: Greek, Latin, and Hebrew. Although classics is a rarefied field with ever-dwindling teaching resources, there was no shortage of Latin instruction at the college. Hebrew, however, was another story, and I could not find a professor with the time or inclination to teach me the language of the Old Testament. So I had to improvise.

I called a local synagogue and investigated language courses on tape. I spent time at the library perusing a decaying nineteenth-century Hebrew grammar and started teaching myself the alphabet, training my eyes to read from right to left. I hounded the one member of the religion faculty, Miriam Dean-Otting, who might have been able to help, with the hope of conveying my unflagging passion and dedication. And just when I thought that I had exhausted all possible options and was about to give up, a door opened and a master appeared.

One afternoon, I received an unexpected phone call from Professor Dean-Otting. She said that an emeritus professor, Dr. Eugen Kullmann, might be able to take me on as a student, but I would need to go and meet with him first, to see if I was a good fit. As an undergraduate at Kenyon in the 1970s, she had studied with Dr. Kullmann and knew firsthand the level of commitment he required of his students. Her tone of voice conveyed a cautious optimism, tempered by the possibility that after meeting me, Dr. Kullmann might not be inclined to move forward with the independent study.

Dr. Kullmann lived about a mile from campus in a neglected little house on a bucolic hill on the other side of a narrow river winding through the cornfields. He had recently suffered a stroke that relegated him mostly to his home, and he hadn't taken on a student in more than a decade. But he remained a towering figure in the intellectual life of the college community, a last living remnant of classical European education and erudition that had reached its heights during the late nineteenth century. Rumor had it that Dr. Kullmann knew as many as twenty languages, and according to an apocryphal story, at one point in his career he had taught eleven classes over the course of a single semester in five different departments—classics, psychology, philosophy, German, and religion. Of course, to Dr. Kullmann these academic distinctions were laughably arbitrary, and he often spoke about the importance of playing the "grand piano" of all humanistic disciplines.

As a child, he had been educated in the gymnasium system in Germany and later completed his undergraduate and graduate work in Basel, Switzerland, studying under luminaries such as Martin Buber, until moving to the United States in 1946. His house in rural Ohio overflowed with tired, broken furniture and countless stacks of books. Over the stairwell leading to his musty basement library, a fading poster of Albert Einstein loomed larger than life. And within easy reach of his dining room table, on a small set of shelves, sat the complete essays of Ralph Waldo Emerson, the collected Shakespeare, Voltaire's *Candide,* and Gibbon's *The Decline and Fall of the Roman Empire,* among many other volumes that Dr. Kullmann believed essential reading for anyone who claimed to be educated. He had spent much of his life reading and rereading this small, select group of books.

Once when I asked him about his experiences as a young student, he described a class in which all the pupils were expected to memorize and recite large sections of Homer's *Odyssey* in ancient Greek. The students were seated in order of their rank, and when one of the students at the front of the room made even the smallest of mistakes in his recitation, the instructor would cut him off swiftly by saying, "I'm sorry, but you have no promise," and point him to the back of the room.

I vividly remember the day I submitted myself to a forty-five-minute interview at Dr. Kullmann's home, sweating straight through the armpits of a secondhand Harris Tweed jacket as he reviewed my feeble academic qualifications at his dining room table. Inspecting me through black Coke-bottle glasses, which exponentially magnified the appearance of his bottomless black pupils, he appeared to look straight through me.

"In the olden days," he rumbled, "we began our studies of Latin in what you call elementary school, Greek in what you call middle school, and if we were promising students, Hebrew in high school. You have only one year of Greek and no Latin. What makes you think that you are qualified to study Hebrew?"

His questioning continued in this fashion for at least another thirty minutes, as he depicted the many challenges of Hebrew grammar and pronunciation, implying in not-so-subtle ways that I shouldn't waste my time pursuing something so far out of reach. Apparently he had conducted his own background check prior to my arriving, ascertaining from my Greek professor, Bill McCulloh, that I was a disciplined student with atrocious handwriting who probably struggled with, in McCulloh's words, "a mild, undiagnosed dyslexia." I don't think I said very much during the interview, but I never broke eye contact and listened intently to his every word. In Greek, "to speak well," or *euphemi,* from which we derive the word *euphemism,* also means "to be silent." This much I knew. There was little I could say to sway him, as he had obviously already made up his mind.

Near the end of his disparaging and remarkably compelling effort to convince me to abandon all ambition of becoming a philologist, after he finally seemed to have expended all possible arguments, he leaned closer, paused, and said: "But . . . if you are willing to endure the hardships that we will undertake together, I would be delighted to have one last student." That was the day my true education began.

For three years I visited Dr. Kullmann several days each week to study classical languages and engage in the type of broad, humanistic discourse that I had only dreamed of when I enrolled in college. I had always been a slow reader. When I was a high school student, to my great embarrassment, my parents enrolled me in a speed-reading course, hoping it would result in a much-needed bump in my SAT scores. However, at Dr. Kullmann's house I learned to read even more slowly.

Most mornings, regardless of the weather, I would walk down a steep, winding hill, past oxidizing trestles and undulating cornfields, up another hill, to his listing one-story house, so overgrown with ferns and untended trees that it was nearly invisible from the road. At the beginning of each lesson, we would spread out four versions of the Old Testament on the table—Hebrew, Greek, Latin, and German—along with lexicons, commentaries, and concordances. Then we would proceed to read five lines in five hours, stopping often to scrutinize prepositions, idioms, and potential errors of transcription, while comparing translations and digressing, sometimes for hours, to investigate the etymologies of words. The name for this meticulous cross-textual method of reading, almost completely lost to the secular world, is *exegesis,* a Greek word that means "to lead out" or "lead out from." Rather than scanning for surface-level comprehension, as quickly and efficiently as possible, the goal is to extract layers upon layers of significance through careful analysis and interpretation.

As we moved through Jonah and sections of Amos and Ecclesiastes, and later sections of Virgil's *Aeneid*, portions of the Homeric epics, Euripides's *Alcestis*, Saint Augustine's *Confessions*, and Goethe's *Faust*, Dr. Kullmann would break up the sessions with provocative questions.

"What is the job of the philologist?" he once asked, and then before I could respond, he answered, "When W. H. Auden was asked by Barbara Walters in a *20/20* interview why he wrote poetry, he replied: 'To save the words.' That is also the job of the philologist."

I quickly discovered that loving words, in the true sense of philology, meant salvaging some from obscurity, while discarding others that were, as Dr. Kullmann often said, "as abused as library books." I jettisoned words such as *interesting* (in Latin, "to be between") and *nice* (in Latin, "ignorance") from my vocabulary, and I developed a reverence for words like *enthusiasm* (in Greek, "possession by a god") and *magnanimous* (in Latin, "big soul"). I learned that the Greeks had at least three verbs that meant "to love," each with its own subtle shades of meaning: affection between friends and family members, erotic love, unconditional love. The Hebrews believed the seat of emotion, *nephesh*, resided in the throat, while the Greeks cataloged countless centers of emotion and cognition, ranging from the soul to the mind to organs for which there is no corollary today, including the *thumos*, which resides in the chest and guides certain kinds of decision making.

I learned many things during my sessions with Dr. Kullmann, but perhaps the most important was to relate what I was reading in classical texts to events in the contemporary world. One of the requirements of studying with him was coming prepared to discuss the news. We treated this daily exchange of current events as an integral part of each session, connecting the ancient mythological past to the morning's headlines. I vividly remember the day *The New York Times* replaced its time-honored black-and-white layout with a large color photo on the front page, top of the fold. Judging from Dr. Kullmann's reaction that morning, Western civilization had abruptly come to an end.

At Dr. Kullmann's home, reading meant working methodically, patiently through a text, forging connections across languages, cultures, religions, and time. However, it also meant stepping back from the text to digest what it said. "What is the secret to reading?" he would often ask, with a slightly mischievous smile. "In the olden days, we would read a passage from a text, then close the book, and smoke a pipe or a cigarette and think 'What have I just read?' But you do not smoke, do you, Dr. Bryan?" he would playfully inquire.

"The secret of reading is to close the book."

Over the course of my studies at Kenyon, both with Dr. Kullman and in other classes, I found myself returning to one particular book, Aristotle's *Poetics*, in order to deepen my understanding of Greek tragedy and how the ancient world might have viewed it. Aristotle divides the plots of tragedies into simple and complex structures. In a complex tragedy, the plot hinges and then swings upon the one-two punch of what he calls *anagnorisis*, "recognition," and *peripeteia*, "reversal." In such tragedies, a protagonist moves decisively in one direction (Oedipus, the king of Thebes, searches tirelessly for the murderer of King Laius), but upon making an earth-shattering discovery (Oedipus is himself the murderer for whom he is searching, the pollution that is plaguing his land, as well as the incestuous lover of his own mother), he takes an abrupt turn in a new direction (Oedipus gouges out his eyes and walks off into the desert in self-imposed exile). In this depiction of human behavior, an ancient psychology begins to emerge, one that is concerned with human insight and the logical connection between actions and their consequences.

Aristotle also argues that one of the most important elements of Greek tragedy is "suffering." By portraying physical pain and emotional anguish, tragedies were designed to elicit powerful emotions. But how, and to what end? Tragedies, by portraying well-intentioned people passing rapidly from prosperity to affliction, evoke "pity and fear." Pity, because we all make mistakes. Fear, because the suffering portrayed in ancient Greek tragedy is horrifying and extreme.

The goal of eliciting these emotions, Aristotle argues, is to bring about *catharsis*. Thousands upon thousands of pages have been written about what he intended by this one word, which in ancient Greek means "to cleanse, purify, refine," but none of these words in English fully conveys the spirit of what Aristotle may have intended, or for that matter the experience of ancient audiences. All well-balanced people feel healthy amounts of pity and fear, when appropriate. So I take Aristotle's *catharsis* to mean "the purification of potentially dangerous emotions, such as pity and fear, of their toxicity," rather than "the complete eradication of these emotions."

The philosopher Plato was no fan of Greek tragedy: he banned all tragic poets and "the rest of the imitative tribe" from the utopian city he described in *The Republic*, his treatise on the ideal state. The main character, based on Plato's great master, Socrates, states in Book 10 that "all poetical imitations are ruinous to the understanding of the hearers" and later concludes that if the "honeyed muse" is allowed to enter the city, the state will be ruled not by reason and law but by "pleasure and pain."

In Plato's assessment, imitation, or *mimesis,* is dangerously removed from the truth of reality. And tragedy, the most developed and persuasive form of *mimesis,* arouses aberrant emotions that cloud our ability to reason and hasten the disintegration of a just society. Tragedy aimed to sweep audiences away—emotionally and physically—with powerful performances, encouraging spectators to indulge in the perilous activity of setting aside reason and being overwhelmed with emotions. This is what made tragedy, in Plato's view, so corrosively and insidiously dangerous for the state. It was inherently manipulative, as well as an enemy to reason and skepticism.

Plato's suspicious view of tragedy influenced generations of scholars, and by the late nineteenth century, a pathological interpretation of the word *catharsis* had become widely accepted in academic circles, one that depicted pity and fear as unhealthy, destructive emotions. As we have seen, Aristotle contends in *The Poetics* that the purpose of tragedy is to arouse pity and fear not for the sake of simply arousing them, or in service of mere entertainment, but in order to purify or refine them of their toxic qualities.

I would add that perhaps tragedy aimed to arouse powerful responses, including pity and fear, in order to facilitate a healthy and balanced response to personal suffering and the suffering of others. The Greeks championed the philosophical concept *sophrosyne,* or "healthy, balanced mind," epitomized by moderation, temperance, and self-control. Perhaps tragedy was a means of reestablishing *sophrosyne* in the Athenian populace, which for whatever reasons—repeated exposure to war, pestilence, or death—had careened off balance; perhaps it was a ritualized and communal method of mitigating the cumulative effects of chronic stress and prolonged exposure to trauma.

In 1993 a team of psychologists at Yale coined the term *allostatic load* to refer to the physical strain of the body's stress response—hormones such as epinephrine and cortisol—upon the cardiovascular system and other organs and tissues. The more exposure one has to acute stressors, the more unbalanced the autonomic nervous system becomes. Maybe tragedy was a mass therapy for lowering the Athenian allostatic load and recalibrating the city's response to stress. On any given day during the City Dionysia, the annual spring theater festival and religious holiday at which Attic tragedies were performed, nearly a third of the citizens in Athens would have been present to watch the tragedies, as a community. By bringing about catharsis, purifying Athenians of toxic levels of stress hormones, the tragedies restored balance—*sophrosyne*—to the autonomic nervous systems of individual citizens as well as to the body politic of Athens.

Aristotle's use of the word *catharsis* suggests that tragedies were designed to elicit powerful emotional, biochemical, and physiological responses from audiences. If tragedy, in fact, aims to arouse and then purify emotions—such as pity and fear—then rather than posing an insidious and corrosive threat to the health of the individual and the state, as Plato thought, tragedy was, and is, a powerful tool for positive change, one whose vast and untapped potential for propagating healthy responses to stress remains wholly underestimated.

III

Over spring break my senior year, I remained on campus after it had emptied of students and enlisted a handful of friends to help construct a makeshift amphitheater on the side of a gently sloping hill in front of an abandoned horse stable, next to one of the dining halls. I was attempting to replicate the Theater of Dionysus, the ancient amphitheater that still sits on the south slope of the Athenian acropolis. We purchased plywood from a local lumberyard and built a dozen long, narrow benches, which we drove into the soft, rain-soaked earth with rubber mallets. The dilapidated stable served as the *skene,* the building that stood behind the stage in many ancient Greek amphitheaters, and a raised wooden platform at the bottom of the hill set the playing area apart from the *orchestra,* a semicircular patch of earth where members of the chorus would dance and sing.

We rented a light board and some Par Cans from a theatrical supply store in Columbus, Ohio, and hung the lights from towering metal pipes, as well as from trees. Though it was certainly a gamble to stage anything outdoors in April, let alone at night, given the likelihood of rain, winds, and plummeting temperatures, it was the latest in the semester that I could feasibly push the production before final exams and graduation.

For my senior project, I had written a new translation of Euripides's *Bacchae,* a play that dramatizes the arrival of Dionysus—the god of wine, ecstasy, and intoxication—in the ancient city of Thebes, and portrays the wide swath of destruction left in his path. The play premiered at the Theater of Dionysus in 405 BC, after Euripides's death.

In the play, Dionysus first comes to Thebes in the form of a charismatic preacher who sends the local women out of their homes and into the hills dancing in ecstatic frenzy for the new god. He then spars with an untested king, a puritanical young man—an *ephebe,* or late adolescent—named Pentheus, who attempts to imprison the "preacher" and his foreign followers, the Bacchants, for inciting disorder in the city. At the end of the play, in a particularly gruesome scene, King Pentheus dies at the hands of his own mother, Agaue, who hunts him down and, along with her sisters, rips him to pieces with her bare hands in a hallucinatory state, mistaking him for a mountain lion. In the span of one day, the seemingly indiscriminate violence of the god of intoxication levels Thebes, sparing no one.

As the culminating event of my time in college, I directed a fully realized production of the *Bacchae* in that ersatz theater. I conscripted a motley assortment of philosophy, anthropology, classics, and religion majors to perform it, along with the local hippie drum circle, replete with tom-toms, African *djembes,* and an Australian didgeridoo, a low vibratory tubelike instrument that we employed at key moments to underscore the numinous presence of the god.

In ancient productions of Greek tragedies, actors portraying Olympian gods were often hoisted on a towering crane, or *deus ex machina* ("god from machine"), high above the Athenian crowd in order to deliver dramatic speeches at the end. In my production, a low-riding light-blue Buick Skylark was to serve that function. When the god appeared in his divine form at the end of the play, he was to slowly roll into the orchestra with a throng of Bacchants bouncing in the backseat to the bump and thrum of low bass tones, vibrating through black-tinted windows.

As luck would have it, on opening night, minutes before the audience began to arrive, the actor playing Dionysus got stoned and accidentally locked his keys inside the *machina,* which happened to be parked directly in front of the stage, rather than behind the stable, where it belonged. I had to call AAA to have a tow truck driver come shock open the electric locks so that we could start on time. Thankfully we did.

The audience arrived and huddled under wool blankets, smoking cigarettes and passing around jugs of cheap red wine, shivering in the frigid night air and illuminated by the flickering, ambient light of tiki torches. The performers quickly recovered from their rocky start, and as the Bacchants danced, hoping to bring the ancient play to life for an audience of young revelers, they tossed glittery Mardi Gras necklaces into the crowd and pulled audience members up to dance in the aisles to the swelling rhythms of the drum circle. With full-throated intensity, they stormed the stage and drove the action of the play barreling forward, careening from moments of levity, irony, and gallows humor. The crowd responded with hoots and hollers, whistles and jeers, uproarious laughter, catcalls, and cries of delight and horror, as the ragtag company of amateur actors shredded their vocal cords and rolled in the mud. Finally came the act of unthinkable violence, when Pentheus's mother and sisters pull him down from a tree and decapitate him. The audience fell silent.

Later that night, around three a.m., as I sat in the

window of my one-room apartment in the center of town, I listened to stumbling-drunk coeds calling and responding across campus with ancient Greek choral passages from Euripides's play, imitating the ecstatic shouts—or *ololuges*—of Bacchants dancing for Dionysus.

Staging the *Bacchae* in rural Ohio solidified—once and for all—my decision not to pursue an academic career, for it was in directing Euripides's play and hearing the audience react that I first began to comprehend the text. With unprecedented clarity, I suddenly knew what I wanted to do with my life. Though it was sobering, after several years of intense study, to realize that I would not be a philologist, at least not in the traditional sense, I had discovered in the process of directing that I was better suited for staging Greek drama than for analyzing it from behind a desk.

No one gets closer to words, and to the impulses behind them, than actors and directors working intensely on a play. The main difference between a translator and a director, when it comes to performed texts, is that a translator has only words at his disposal, while a director can employ the entire theatrical palette of lights, movement, sound, costumes, speech/diction, and bodies moving through space in order to transform words on a page into a production on a stage. As I worked on Euripides's *Bacchae,* I soon came to realize that I was a director and a translator—an intermediary between ancient plays and audiences—and that directing and translating were one and the same.

The difference between an exhilarating production of a classical play and a bloodless museum piece depends on how the director approaches the text. Sometimes being respectful of an ancient playwright's intentions means finding forms through which his plays may thrive in the contemporary world. Each successive generation, from the Roman tragedian Seneca—whose influence cannot be overestimated—to the tragedians of the Italian and English Renaissance to the present, has reinvented ancient Greek tragedy, usually in its own image. The secret to understanding tragedy and to helping it reach audiences today, I discovered, is to close the book and reimagine it for our time.

IV

Friedrich Nietzsche's main argument in *We Philologists* is that the ancient world is often introduced to young students "as if they were well-informed and matured men." He argues that "we are forced to concern ourselves with antiquity at a wrong period of our lives," and he concludes that only "at the end of the twenties, its meaning begins to dawn on one." When I was twenty-six, I experienced a life-altering event that fundamentally changed my relationship with antiquity. It was in the years that followed that the significance of Greek tragedy began to dawn on me.

While in college, over the summers, I worked as a counselor at the University of Virginia Young Writers Workshop, a camp for precocious, motivated teenagers who are serious about writing. It was there that I met

Laura, whose story I touched upon in the prologue. She was an eighteen-year-old poet with cystic fibrosis (CF), a genetic disorder that disrupts the body's ability to regulate sweat, digestive fluids, and mucus—affecting the lungs, sinuses, intestines, liver, and pancreas, among many other organs. Laura had a bright, beautiful smile, knowing eyes, rosy cheeks, long elegant arms and legs, and hunched shoulders, all characteristics that I later came to associate with the disease. Her unmistakably raspy voice and tubercular-sounding cough seemed to accompany her everywhere she went, along with a wicked and—at times—blistering sense of humor.

Laura had been diagnosed with CF at three days old, which in the early 1980s was most certainly a death sentence. CF is still treated on the pediatric side of hospitals because so few patients live to see early adulthood. The median life expectancy has crept higher each year—it is now in the low thirties—with advancements in antibiotics and surgical treatments, including lung transplants. However, as of today there is no cure, just stopgaps against the inevitable.

CF is caused by a genetic mutation, one that primarily affects Caucasians; in order for a baby to be born with CF, both of the parents must carry the gene. Today a routine blood test is administered to screen at-risk populations, but at the time Laura was born, this type of genetic screening was not as prevalent. In the end, no one was more crushed by the news of Laura's diagnosis than her father, Jon, a gifted physician who immediately understood its implications.

The summer I met Laura was oppressively hot for Charlottesville, Virginia, a bucolic university town nestled in the foothills of the Blue Ridge Mountains. Temperatures soared well into the nineties, and the humidity hovered around 100 percent. Because people with CF are unable to perspire in order to cool themselves down, they can easily overheat. Also, poor air quality can quickly compromise their ability to breathe. This meant that Laura had to be driven to and from class and appointments at the hospital, and for a few weeks I had the privilege of being her chauffeur.

Laura was the kind of person who, aware of her mortality from an early age, did not waste words. As anyone who spent more than twenty minutes with her can attest, she invariably moved, even with strangers, straight from small talk to the big questions, and she wasn't afraid to openly discuss illness or death. As her driver, I quickly learned much of her life story, how she had grown up dividing her time between her parents' apartment on the Upper East Side of Manhattan and a pediatric unit at Columbia-Presbyterian Medical Center. For many years, the hospital floor had housed a tight-knit group of CF patients who were de facto siblings, as well as close confidants and friends, until it was discovered in the mid-1990s that they were cross-pollinating a harmful bacterium that was hastening their deaths. Laura and her friends were banned from seeing one another, except on rare occasions, such as funerals, of which there would be many in the years that followed.

She had already, at seventeen, endured more physical and emotional challenges than most people see in a lifetime, but rather than focusing on her own discomfort or pain, she mostly concerned herself with the suffering of others. I spent more time telling her my story, while shuttling her around campus in the passenger seat of a white university van, about my father's worsening health due to late-stage diabetes, than hearing hers. It was comforting to talk with someone who was no stranger to chronic illness yet remained spirited and full of life. I certainly didn't comprehend, until many years later, how much of a challenge it had been for her to wake each morning, clear her sinuses, nebulize her lungs, and show up at the poetry workshop with the singular intention of blending in with her peers. I had no idea how hard she worked at seeming normal.

After meeting at the workshop, we stayed in touch through letters and occasional e-mails. I enrolled in an MFA directing program in California with the intention of staging more Greek and Roman plays, while she completed her final year at the Chapin School, an elite all-girls school in New York City. The following summer, while visiting New York and subletting a windowless room in the East Village for six weeks, I decided to give her a call, to see how she was doing. We met that night at a café on St. Mark's Place, drank carafes of coffee, and stayed up late into the evening talking and laughing on the roof of a tenement building on East Fifth Street.

Though Laura's health had already begun to decline, she carefully steered the conversation away from her own troubles and zeroed in on mine. At the time, I was conflicted about whether to return to graduate school for two more years or to move to New York to begin my directing career in earnest. Laura listened with the same attention and compassion she would have afforded a dying friend, while I prattled on about my armchair theories regarding ancient Greek tragedy. Nothing romantic transpired, and I distinctly remember feeling a sort of brotherly affection for her and a vague desire to protect her from the unimaginable struggles to come. She encouraged me to return to California and finish what I had started.

I heeded her advice, but before flying back to California in late August, I sent her a letter, along with a copy of Dostoyevsky's *The Brothers Karamazov*, that ended, "Please know that your chauffeur will always be waiting to drive you wherever you need to go."

Over the next two years, while I completed my directing degree out west, Laura fought for time, attempting to live the life of an ordinary college student at Brown University, while waiting for new lungs. This meant, among many things that others her age would have found inconceivable, that she walked to class with an oxygen tank concealed inside her backpack. It meant that when her weight dropped precipitously, she took in supplemental nutrition through a tube in her stomach, just to remain eligible for surgery. It also meant dance parties, drinking games, late-night coed revelry, and fleeting, inebriated hook-ups. Though she had little hope of surviving her twenties—most of her friends who had the disease, the ones she'd grown up with at Columbia-Presbyterian, had already died—Laura had every intention of living like her peers at Brown.

While I was in California, I missed the grueling months leading up to the transplant, as well as the first year of her punishing recovery. One of Laura's defining features was that she left many of the people she met with the lasting impression that they had exchanged something rare and intimate. Yet although I regarded her as a good friend, I was barely involved in her life. Months later, long after her family and many of her closest friends had been thoroughly exhausted by trying to support her through the snowballing challenges she faced after the transplant, I finally came back into her life and learned the story of what had happened since we last saw each other on a rooftop in the East Village. Her recovery had been a roller-coaster ride of unexpected complications, including post-transplant lymphoma, bowel obstructions, and pulmonary infections.

In 2001, when Laura's old lungs began to give out, so riddled with infection that some doctors in New York had ruled them inoperable, she managed to persuade an open-minded transplant surgeon at Boston Children's Hospital to give her a chance at having an adult life, however abbreviated it might turn out to be. The odds were decidedly stacked against her, due to an antibiotic-resistant bacterium that had invaded and set up camp in her body, but Laura nonetheless received the double lung transplant. And with it came a new lease on life.

When I reconnected with her, shortly after moving

to New York in January 2002, she was breathing at
95 percent capacity. On an unseasonably warm winter
night, she came to visit me in Brooklyn, where I was subletting a small studio. We walked close to five miles,
from the Hasidic neighborhood under the Williamsburg
Bridge to the postindustrial ruins of Greenpoint, stopping at bars and restaurants and taking in the soaring
Manhattan skyline from a seawall along the East River.
She seemed more vibrant, more full of energy and hope
than I had ever seen her, bounding through cobblestone
streets upon stiltlike legs, laughing with full-throated
abandon at her own jokes. It was as if, for a brief moment, she had been cured.

Later that spring I took an Amtrak train from Penn
Station to Providence, to visit her at Brown. When she
picked me up at the train station, I could immediately
tell, simply by the way her shoulders curled and by the
strain with which she coughed and walked, that something had changed. Looking at her from a distance, as
she waited for me in the lobby of the train station at the
top of the escalator, I had the impression that she had
aged twenty years in two and a half months.

That same winter she had been visited by a wave of
debilitating panic attacks. Fits of shaking would over-
whelm her entire body until in some instances she would
stop breathing for a few minutes and then, miraculously,
begin again, with no external assistance, as if she were
dying and then waking from death. The doctors did not
know what to make of it. Some dismissed the episodes
as psychosomatic in nature and upped her dosages of

antianxiety medications. Others characterized the episodes as "drug-seeking" behavior, accusing her of deliberately staging the fits in order to be prescribed more medications. By this point, though, Laura was off the medical charts, floating in pharmaceutical outer space. There was no clear explanation for her fits, no precedent or research for doctors to draw upon when treating her. In many ways, she was on her own.

During that brief visit to Brown, we stumbled clumsily into a borderless romance, which would span the remaining year of Laura's life. From the moment we first kissed, awkwardly, hesitantly, in her apartment, I knew I would soon face a choice, one that would define my own moral character and perhaps the rest of my life. If I truly cared for Laura, then I would put everything else on hold and live up to the pledge to drive her wherever she needed to go. But a nagging and persistent voice of self-preservation within me said to run away, as fast as I could. I tried my best to ignore the voice and simply follow my instincts, but the voice grew louder the closer we became. We were at different points in our lives—she still in college and I just starting out in New York—and so living up to my promise would mean patiently waiting until she was ready for my help, but also jumping into action when the time came. In spite of my better judgment, I had fallen in love with her, and when the moment arrived when she truly needed me, there really wasn't much of a choice to make.

Laura finished out the spring semester at Brown and started a summer internship working for the New York

State Office of Children and Family Services, shadowing social workers in the outer boroughs of New York City making apartment visits in housing projects. Over the spring and summer months, her health continued to flag, but she remained committed to writing about her experiences—in and out of the hospital—and to pursuing a professional career helping disadvantaged children. In August 2002 the National Public Radio program *All Things Considered* ran an audio diary that Laura had recorded in the months leading up to and following her double lung transplant, called "My So-Called Lungs." The broadcast garnered her a great deal of positive attention, and soon, with the help of a literary agent, she received a book contract from Hyperion for a manuscript she had drafted in a class at Brown about living with CF and surviving her lung transplant. In short order, Laura was accomplishing much of what she had set out to do in the time she had left.

Soon after she returned to Brown that fall, a well-intentioned doctor informed her that her lungs were in the early stages of rejection and that she probably had less than six months to live. He encouraged her to think about how she would like to spend her remaining time. Aspiring to be a normal college student suddenly lost its appeal. Later that week, with the help of her father and one of his friends, Laura packed up her apartment in Providence and drove back to New York to die. Before she left, she called me with the news. She did not want her parents to have to care for her during the last months of her life, as she couldn't bear the thought of burdening them with her death or, for that matter, of dying in her childhood bedroom. She wanted to use her book advance to spend her final months living an independent adult existence and asked if I would help her find an apartment and see things through to the end.

Three days before she died, Laura awoke from a narcotized, thirty-six-hour slumber, waved me over to her side of the bed, lifted her oxygen mask, which had been precariously rigged by her father to pump fifteen liters of oxygen per minute into her failing lungs, and said, "There's this tugboat circling for me in the river, and I was wondering if you were planning on getting on it?"

It was the middle of March. The winter—one of the harshest on record in New York City—had finally begun to thaw, and the trees in Union Square, two blocks from our loft on Thirteenth Street, were sprouting small red buds. Spring was in the air, and the vernal equinox was fast approaching, a moment between seasons when the earth ceases dying and begins to be reborn. I had read somewhere that some ancient cultures believed that the greatest among us, the heroes, always died on the equinox. As I watched Laura approach death, it occurred to me that perhaps this was because heroes squeezed everything from life until the last possible moment.

In the four months since we'd moved in together, Laura and I had attempted to wring as much from life as humanly possible. In December, when she had required just a few liters of oxygen to traverse the block, we would go see experimental plays in the East Village or out to dinner at nearby restaurants. On New Year's Eve we chartered a cruise at Chelsea Piers for a hundred of her friends and watched the fireworks light up the icy waters surrounding the Statue of Liberty at midnight. In January, as her walking became more labored and she became increasingly dependent upon higher levels of oxygen just to sit up in an armchair and converse, we hosted raucous, late-night dinner parties, drinking through a case of red wine over a few weeks. Some evenings she would rally and remain at the table for hours, regaling us all with jokes and stories. Other nights she would simply listen from her bed to the ambient sounds of people talking well into the night. Either way, she didn't wish to wait until her memorial service to gather all the people who were important to her in one place. In fact, she wasn't interested in mourning at all. She wanted to celebrate the gift of her existence.

In early February, in honor of her twenty-second birthday, we held a high tea in the apartment, with finger sandwiches and delicate French pastries, for all her Chapin School friends and, later that same night, an intimate dinner for a handful of those who remained closest near the end. In the three weeks that followed, Laura would see nearly every remaining person in her life and gently, lovingly say goodbye.

By early March, the steady stream of visitors slowed to a trickle. Laura's energy began to fade, along with her will to live. Due to a heavy load of opiates that helped ease her immense discomfort, she spent more of her days, by this point, asleep than awake. By the second week of March, she had stopped eating (with the exception of mini marzipan-chocolate cakes that I brought her from a local bakery) and rarely drank water. Her long, slender frame had wasted away to less than eighty pounds.

Whenever she awoke, it was usually in a semihallucinatory state in which she would say things that, due to drug-induced amnesia, I would have to remind her of later. The day she asked me about the "tugboat" circling for her in the river was no exception.

"Can you tell me more about the river?" I asked.

"It's the Hudson," she said, widening her eyes as if to indicate that I, of all people, should understand the mythological allusion.

"I'm sorry," I quietly replied, moving a strand of her hair away from her eyes. "I won't be getting on. This is as far as I go. But you definitely should. It's time."

Three days later Laura woke up, unstrapped her oxygen mask, and set it quietly on the pillow beside her. The nurse asked all of us who were present—her mother, father, her friend Abby, and me—to gather around the bed. Laura held her mother's hand.

It took roughly twenty minutes for her breathing to become labored, but all the while she remained acutely, fearlessly conscious, comforting us individually and collectively with gentle words. "It's okay," she repeated softly to each of us, especially to her grieving father, who was not prepared to lose his darling girl that day. "It's okay."

In the last seconds, as she gasped violently for air in long involuntary bursts, with the rattle of death in her final breaths, and using what remained of her inimitable voice, she tenderly repeated, "I love you. I love you. I love you. I love you," as the force that animated her slipped quietly from her body in one final exhalation.

Laura died at eight p.m. on March 20, 2003—the exact moment of the vernal equinox.

Although I wasn't aware of it at the time, witnessing Laura's graceful death opened my eyes to what the Greek tragedies I had studied in school were trying to convey. Through tragedy, the great Athenian poets were not articulating a pessimistic or fatalistic view of human existence; nor were they bent on filling audiences with despair. Instead, they were giving voice to timeless human experiences—of suffering and grief— that, when viewed by a large audience that had shared those experiences, fostered compassion, understanding, and a deeply felt interconnection. Through tragedy, the Greeks faced the darkness of human existence as a community.

In the months and years that followed, I saw these ancient stories—filled with conflict, ambivalence, and loss—no longer as subjects of academic study but as lived experience. The extreme emotions that they portrayed now seemed like a natural extension of my own.

If ancient Greek tragedies could speak directly to me, or could capture the essence of something private and seemingly unknowable, such as the death of someone I loved, then they could also speak to anyone who had lived—in some direct way—the human experiences they describe.

PTSD IS FROM BC

I

Picture thousands of citizen-soldiers seated in an amphitheater on the south slope of the Acropolis in the ancient city of Athens. It's the early spring of 409 BC, and for more than twenty years the Greeks have been fighting a war on multiple fronts against indefatigable adversaries, the Spartans.

The theater rumbles with footsteps as the men climb the aisles to find their seats. At daybreak, the countless rows resound with the powerful blast of a trumpet, signaling the beginning of the City Dionysia, that festival of dramatic performances: three days of plays written and performed by combat veterans, for large audiences of combat veterans.

Today's tragedies were written by a retired general named Sophocles, now in his late eighties. He had been elected general twice during his long tenure in the Athenian army and still carries on his shoulders the unbearable weight of the countless men he led into battle who never returned. He has secretly dedicated the plays to them.

The crowd suddenly silences, as the entire army leaps to its feet in one fluid movement, while ten commanding generals progress to the front of the theater to take their seats in appointed thrones. Behind them the audience is tightly packed. Soldiers stand at attention, shoulder to shoulder, according to tribe, which is their military unit, and according to rank. The hoplite cadets are squeezed into the nosebleed section in the very back, from which the generals now look diminutive, like stick figures placed in front of a quarter-inch model.

Though it's hard to make it out from the rear of the theater, a solemn religious ceremony has begun, a funereal rite. The armor of the war dead is being bestowed upon their bereaved children, who walk slowly to the center of the orchestra, their shoulders sunk, their heads bowed. There is hardly a dry eye in the house as the war orphans—now wards of the polis—collect their fallen fathers' shields. The Athenians have lost thousands of men already this year to war, yet they've had no time to grieve their losses, no sanctioned occasion on which to express the fullness of their emotions, no safe place to scream . . . until now.

The actor playing Philoctetes—a warrior abandoned by his own troops on a desolate island on account of a mysterious illness—soon takes the stage, crawls out of his cave, opens his throat, and begins to wail. He wails for himself. He wails for his friends. He wails for the war dead and their children, and most of all he wails for the warriors who are watching him wail.

He is wailing on their behalf.

When I first told friends that I wanted to present my translations of ancient Greek tragedies to infantry soldiers and Marines on military bases throughout the United States, they looked at me with bewilderment and concern. I suppose at the time it sounded a bit unrealistic, or perhaps just ill advised. Though many scholars had made the connection between ancient Greek drama and Athenian military culture, no one had attempted to perform these plays for active-duty service members, let alone with the hope that they would reveal something timeless and profound about the experience of war.

As a child I knew almost no one in the military. Aside from the movies I had watched, the video games I had played, and the stories I had read in newspapers and in books, I had no regular contact with military culture. My grandfather had served in the navy during World War II, trained as a naval aviator in 1945 but never deployed. The bomb was dropped, and he came home without a scratch and with no memorable war stories to pass on to his grandchildren. My father got an exemption from Vietnam by going to graduate school. Simply put, as a child, I had no idea what military service was, nor any point of reference that would help me understand it.

My ignorance was particularly striking in that my childhood home, Newport News, Virginia, was surrounded by bases: Fort Eustis, Langley Air Force Base,

Naval Amphibious Base Little Creek, Naval Weapons Station Yorktown, Naval Medical Center Portsmouth, and Camp Peary (the training grounds for the CIA). The city was also home to the second-largest privately owned shipyard in the world, where many nuclear submarines, aircraft carriers, and warships were constructed each year. The entire economy was driven and supported by the military-industrial complex, without which, the city would cease to exist.

As a young boy, I grew so accustomed to hearing the sonic booms of screaming F-16 fighter jets over our roof that I stopped hearing them, the way I have now stopped hearing the police and ambulance sirens outside my windows in Brooklyn. Although I lived among service members and veterans—they cut my hair at the barbershop, taught earth science and Spanish at my prep school, and coached my little league baseball team—the military was foreign to me. It was background noise. Like most of the people I knew, I thought of myself as, in principle, against war and, in theory, supportive of veterans.

Then in February 18, 2007, I read a story in *The Washington Post* about the Walter Reed scandal. The damning investigative report described how wounded soldiers returned from Iraq and Afghanistan to substandard, negligent care at our nation's flagship army hospital. Only then did I begin to pay attention to the struggles of returning combat veterans and their families. The article, by staff writers Dana Priest and Anne Hull, began:

Behind the door of Army Spec. Jeremy Duncan's room, part of the wall is torn and hangs in the air, weighted down with black mold. When the wounded combat engineer stands in his shower and looks up, he can see the bathtub on the floor above through a rotted hole. The entire building, constructed between the world wars, often smells like greasy carry-out. Signs of neglect are everywhere: mouse droppings, belly-up cockroaches, stained carpets, cheap mattresses. . . .

The common perception of Walter Reed is of a surgical hospital that shines as the crown jewel of military medicine. But 5½ years of sustained combat have transformed the venerable 113-acre institution into something else entirely—a holding ground for physically and psychologically damaged outpatients. Almost 700 of them—the majority soldiers, with some Marines—have been released from hospital beds but still need treatment or are awaiting bureaucratic decisions before being discharged or returned to active duty.

They suffer from brain injuries, severed arms and legs, organ and back damage, and various degrees of post-traumatic stress. Their legions have grown so exponentially—they outnumber hospital patients at Walter Reed 17 to 1—that they take up every available bed on post and spill into dozens of nearby hotels and apartments leased by the Army.

As I read further in the article, I suddenly became conscious of my willful ignorance. In an effort to ethically distance myself from the wars, I had largely ignored stories about returning service members and veterans, but that position, I would soon discover, was completely untenable. Incensed by the mistreatment of soldiers and their families by the very administration that had sent them to Iraq and Afghanistan, I began thinking about what I could do to raise awareness about the needs of veterans and their families and perhaps rally more people to pay attention.

But I wasn't a psychologist, a social worker, a minister, or a journalist. I was just an aspiring theater director and an amateur classicist with an abiding love for ancient Greek plays. Rather than a fully formed idea, my impulse to present readings of ancient Greek tragedies for combat veterans was what the great stage director Peter Brook has called "a formless hunch." The article about Walter Reed Army Medical Center sent me back to the ancient tragedies on my shelf in search of stories that could bridge the ancient and contemporary worlds and perhaps provide relief to those who were suffering from timeless wounds.

Sophocles's *Philoctetes* is a play about a Greek warrior who, on his way to the Trojan War, is bitten by a poisonous snake and, after contracting a chronic illness, is abandoned for nine long years on a desolate island by his own troops. Willing himself to survive, believ-

ing he is suffering for a reason, he sleeps in a cave, for-
ages for food, and scavenges for herbs to dull the pain
of his wound, all the while hoping that he will one day
be rescued.

However, no one comes to get Philoctetes off the
island, at least not until the Greeks learn from a Trojan seer—nine years later—that they need him and his
invincible bow to win the Trojan War. But by then it's
too late. Years of isolation have reduced him to the
state of an animal and stripped him of his humanity,
his ability to socialize with others and to trust the very
men who have, at long last, come to save him. In spite
of overwhelming bouts of unbearable pain, Philoctetes
refuses to accept medical treatment from the army and
the nation that betrayed him.

PHILOCTETES
Imagine my surprise
when I awoke, the tears
I shed, the sound of my
sadness. All of the ships
in the fleet had vanished.

Alone with my infection,
I knew only pain. Time
demanded that I scavenge
for food with this sacred
bow, which saved my life.
I would crawl through deep
mud on stiff knees, scraping

my rotten foot against rocks.
When water was scarce, I
survived by collecting ice.
I spent cold winter nights
without fire, but rubbing
stones together for their spark,
I saved myself from certain death.

So you see. I have everything
I need here in this cave, except
a cure for my endless affliction.

As I read about Walter Reed and saw photographs
in national newspapers of American soldiers waiting
for treatment in understaffed hospitals, it occurred to
me that through modern medicine we had developed
the ability to save the lives of more soldiers than ever
before. Roughly 95 percent of the injured service members who lived long enough to receive medical treatment
would survive their injuries and return to the States to
begin the long road to recovery. Due to major medical
advancements, more than thirty thousand veterans of
the wars in Iraq and Afghanistan sustained and survived moderate to penetrating traumatic brain injuries
(TBIs), sometimes accompanied by multiple amputa-
tions and other complex wounds that would have been
fatal during any previous conflict.

However, by saving so many lives, we had also
refined our ability to prolong the agony and isolation of
wounded soldiers, like Philoctetes, stranded on islands

of chronic illness. We were creating a vast subclass of profoundly injured veterans who would be dependent on the care of others for decades to come.

Over the previous year, I had directed several readings of my translation of *Philoctetes* at venues in New York City. *Philoctetes* was the first play I had translated after Laura's death. I had been drawn to it because of its vivid depiction of chronic illness and its impact upon patients and caregivers. During those early readings, I had noticed the play's immediate effect on audiences. The performances, which were always raw and powerful, seemed to leave people buzzing in their seats, unsure how to respond to the graphic, unbridled depiction of human suffering at the center of the play, but wishing to talk about it.

After one reading in the basement of the Culture Project, an Off-Broadway theater in the East Village, a doctor contacted me, suggesting that *Philoctetes* might be used to frame conversations about doctor-patient relations at a teaching hospital or medical school. He encouraged me to reach out to the directors of "medical humanities" programs in the city, to see if there might be interest in such a performance.

The first call that I made, at the suggestion of Laura's father, was to a physician named Lyuba Konopasek, who directed medical humanities at Weill Cornell Medical College and—as fate would have it—had recently taught Laura's book, *Breathing for a Living*, to her first-year medical students. Less than three months later, with Lyuba's help, I presented *Philoctetes* at Weill Cornell for an audience of first- and third-year medical students and faculty members. Though few in the audience had heard of the play, many responded strongly—both ethically and emotionally—to it. In the discussion that followed, I was startled to hear medical students and physicians making strikingly candid, insightful connections between the play and their own training and practice, quoting passages from the text and relating them to professional experiences. The play, it seemed, had the power to elicit crucial dialogue about challenging questions surrounding patient care.

An article ran in the health section of *The New York Times* about the Weill Cornell reading. The reporter, Abigail Zuger, described *Philoctetes* as "a case right out of a chronic-care ward in a Veterans Administration hospital." It was around then that I started putting things together, seeing the potential of *Philoctetes* to speak not just to medical audiences but to those who had served in the military. Philoctetes, after all, wasn't just a chronically ill patient. He was a veteran who had been abandoned by the nation that sent him to war. If I could present readings of the play for service members and veterans, like the struggling subjects of the *Post* article, maybe something healing could happen.

I made phone calls and knocked on the doors of military leaders, hoping to convince them that performing ancient Greek plays for their troops would result in crucial conversations about the challenges of returning from war, helping to ease the pain that so many were experiencing back home. I tried to find sympathetic leaders at places such as West Point and Annapolis, where Thucydides and Herodotus were part of the core curriculum, but most, if not all, of the doors were closed in my face, some politely, others not.

That all changed on January 13, 2008. That was the day *The New York Times* published an article entitled "Across America, Deadly Echoes of Foreign Battles," as part of a series about the difficulties faced by returning veterans called "War Torn." With that article, the investigative reporters Deborah Sontag and Lizette Alvarez broke the national story about how the violence from the wars in Iraq and Afghanistan had arrived on American soil. It began with a summation of news headlines:

> Town by town across the country, headlines have been telling similar stories. Lakewood, Wash.: "Family Blames Iraq After Son Kills Wife." Pierre, S.D.: "Soldier Charged with Murder Testifies About Postwar Stress." Colorado Springs: "Iraq War Vets Suspected in Two Slayings, Crime Ring."

Sontag and Alvarez reported that they had verified "121 cases in which veterans of Iraq and Afghanistan committed a killing in this country, or were charged with one, after their return from war." Of those cases, three-quarters involved service members who were still serving when the murders took place.

More than half the killings involved guns,
and the rest were stabbings, beatings,
strangulations and bathtub drownings.
Twenty-five offenders faced murder,
manslaughter or homicide charges for fatal
car crashes resulting from drunken, reckless
or suicidal driving. About a third of the
victims were spouses, girlfriends, children or
other relatives.

On every page of the article, in every paragraph, I saw
writ large the story of Sophocles's *Ajax*, which tells the
story of a fierce Greek warrior who slides into a depression near the end of the Trojan War after losing his close
friend, Achilles. In a berserk rage, Ajax attempts to
murder his commanding officers, fails, and ultimately
takes his own life.

> AJAX
> What should I do now?
>
> The gods hate me,
> the Greeks loathe me,
> the Trojans despise me.
>
> Perhaps I should set
> sail for home, across
> the open sea, leaving
> behind ships and men,
> and the sons of Atreus?

But what will I say
to my father, Telamon,
when he sees my face?

How will he even bear
to look at me when I
explain how I disgraced
our family name for
which he fought so hard?

His heart will break
right then and there.

Should I scale the walls
of Troy and face the army
by myself, show them what
I'm made of, and then die?

No, that would only
please the generals.

I must do something
bold to erase all doubt
in my father's mind
that his son was anything
but a coward.

When a man suffers
without end in sight
and takes no pleasure

in living his life, day
by day wishing for
death, he should not
live out all his years.

It is pitiful when men
hold on to false hopes.

A great man must
live in honor or die
an honorable death.

Ajax, a decorated soldier from a prestigious military family, was considered by many to be the strongest warrior in the Greek army, second only to Achilles.
The Greeks called him "the shield," because he and
his troops always fought in the most dangerous battles and sustained the greatest losses, as they shielded
the rest of the army from the worst attacks. And so
by recounting the story of Ajax, including his bloody
rampage and subsequent suicide, for a largely military
audience during a century in which Athens saw nearly
eighty years of war, Sophocles, the general officer and
playwright, was sending a clear message to everyone
who had served, or who were training to serve: No
one among us is invulnerable to the invisible wounds
of war.

Sophocles was by no means the only Greek tragedian writing about the cost of war. Aeschylus described the challenges of homecoming in *Agamemnon*.

Euripides depicted the psychological toll of war in *Madness of Heracles,* the moral and spiritual dimensions of going to war in *Iphigenia in Aulis,* and the horror of war atrocities in *Trojan Women.* Though it most certainly had not been lost on audiences in his time, the message of Sophocles's *Ajax,* in particular, seemed uncannily fitting for ours. Even the strongest of warriors can be taken down, long after the battle has been lost or won. The violence of war extends far past the battlefield. Not only was psychological injury, it seems, a persistent and universal problem for warriors twenty-five hundred years ago, but—like Americans today—the ancient Greeks also must have struggled with the violence of war, on and off the battlefield.

Later, in the same article, as if by divine providence or fate, in a section entitled "An Ancient Connection," Sontag and Alvarez put the missing pieces together and pointed directly to the person who would help me mount my first military performance:

In an online course for health professionals, Capt. William P. Nash, the combat/operational stress control coordinator for the Marines, reaches back to Sophocles' account of Ajax, who slipped into a depression after the Trojan War, slaughtered a flock of sheep in a crazed state, and then fell on his own sword.

For about a week, I searched for, and finally located, Captain Nash's e-mail address. I quickly drafted my best pitch, crossed my fingers, and hit send.

Less than twenty-four hours later, I received his reply:

Bryan,

Thanks for your e-mail. I am not a Greek scholar by any means, but what I read about Philoctetes on your website seems compelling and very pertinent to our nation and time. I would be very happy to receive a DVD with a reading. My address is below my signature.

I don't know that I could help arrange any readings of Philoctetes in Marine Corps communities for you, but I wonder if you could give a presentation (and short reading) for our next USMC Combat Stress Conference, probably on the first week of May 2008. We have not nailed down the exact dates and location (though we hope to do that soon), but we will probably have the conference in San Diego. I can surely give you 45 minutes in a plenary session (we would expect 500–800 people). What do you think?

Bill

II

Those Marines who attended the first military reading of my translations of Sophocles's *Ajax* and *Philoctetes* in a Hyatt Ballroom in San Diego came on their own volition. They had freely chosen ancient Greek dinner theater over free tickets to a Padres game, and many of them brought their spouses. The bar and buffet in the back of the cavernous room certainly helped draw the crowd, as did the presence of several well-known actors, including Jesse Eisenberg and David Strathairn. But no one who showed up that night had any idea of what was about to happen.

Earlier that morning I had dragged four bleary-eyed New York actors to a seven a.m. plenary session at a conference on "Combat Operational Stress Control" (the Marine Corps' way of talking about PTSD without pathologizing it) to speak—for a few minutes—to nearly seven hundred Marines, to try to persuade them to attend our performance and discussion. I had done some research and had learned that the three bedrock principles and values upon which the Continental Congress had founded the Marines were honor, courage, and commitment.

So when the retired general who was leading the morning session finished his remarks and it was my turn to speak, I stepped onto the stage with some trepidation. Flanked awkwardly on either side by the actors, I cleared my throat and went for broke: "The stories you will hear tonight are about ancient warriors struggling under the weight of nine years of war to maintain their dignity and to uphold their values—honor, courage, and commitment—the same core values that the Marine Corps strives to uphold today. We hope to see you tonight. Thank you for your service."

The conference planners made no promises, and to be honest, I didn't have high hopes for a large turnout. I wasn't worried about whether the plays would resonate with Marines—I was worried that no one would come. I had consciously chosen to present the scenes from Sophocles's plays as simply and straightforwardly as possible, in the form of a table reading, which even in theatrical circles is rarely enticing. But fully staging a Greek tragedy is fraught with risk and highly problematic, especially for new audiences. The last thing I wanted was for the cultural baggage and pretension long associated with Greek tragedy to get in the way of the audience's connection with the stories.

And so by stripping the performance to its bare essentials, by focusing the actors' considerable talents upon the power of the spoken word, and by choosing and adapting key scenes that I believed would speak to the issues at hand, I hoped to deliver the plays in their purest, most efficacious form, while leaving room for the Marines and their spouses to project their memories upon myths from the Trojan War. Also, by presenting an abbreviated selection of scenes that lasted just over an hour, my hope was to leave time for a conversation that would be as potentially charged and powerful as the actors' performances. From the beginning, the discussion was never an afterthought. In many ways, I saw it as the main event. I have always viewed our performances as catalysts for discussions that otherwise would never have occurred. The readings and discussions are one interdependent thing.

A large number of the Marines who showed up that night probably expected to see a fully staged reenactment of the three hundred Spartans bravely standing down the Persian army at the battle of Thermopylae, featuring hack-and-slash swordplay and pyrotechnics. When they discovered four actors in street clothes sitting at a long table in front of microphones, wielding scripts instead of battle-axes or spears, a sizable portion of the audience was visibly disappointed.

But twenty minutes into the performance—as Bill Camp, the fierce New York actor playing Ajax, wailed and screamed about how he wished to kill Odysseus, and finally resolved that "a great man must live in honor, or die an honorable death," before plunging himself upon the enemy's sword—something in the audience seemed to shift.

All the cell phones disappeared. Everyone in the room leaned forward and "locked on," a military term for staring intensely at something or someone without blinking for a preternaturally long period of time. Some Marines rested their heads in their hands, peering through the cracks in their fingers. Others gazed off into the distance, glazed over but fully listening with every fiber of their being. A few wiped tears from their eyes, tightly gripping spouses' hands, while others smirked at certain words with recognition. It was as if these ancient plays had found their intended audience, almost twenty-five hundred years after they had first been performed.

Dr. Jonathan Shay, the MacArthur Award–winning psychiatrist who has spent his life working with Vietnam veterans, has advanced a theory that storytelling, and Greek tragedy in particular, arose and evolved in the Western world from the need to hear and tell the veteran's story. Sophocles was a general in the Athenian army, and the actors in his plays would undoubtedly have been combat veterans. The Trojan War, roughly dated to 1200 BC, likely seemed as distant in memory to fifth-century Athenians as those Athenians now seem to us. Seen through this lens, Sophocles's plays emerge as a powerful tool, an ancient military technology designed to help those who'd been to war make meaning out of their fragmented memories and to evenly distribute the burden of what they brought back from battle upon the shoulders of all Athenians.

"War is the father of all things," wrote the pre-Socratic philosopher Heraclitus. Many of the greatest humanistic achievements of ancient Athens—arguably one of the most militaristic democracies to ever inhabit the earth—were forged in the crucible of constant military conflict. Storytelling, philosophy, art, and war were vitally and inextricably interconnected. Perhaps one of the most overlooked yet crowning achievements of this ancient democracy, from which we have borrowed so much, was the wholesale use of the arts to communalize the experience of war. The Greeks knew that live drama had the power to convey the spirit of an ultimately indescribable experience. Through their plays, Sophocles and his contemporaries, Aeschylus and Euripides, forged a common public vocabulary for openly acknowledging and discussing the impact of war on individuals, families, and communities.

To be an Athenian citizen during the fifth century
BC meant, among other things, that you were male and
served in the military. Unlike America today, in which
less than half of 1 percent of the population has served
in some of the longest wars in our nation's history, Athens demanded compulsory service of its male citizens.
In light of this glaring disparity, in a challenge to readers, Shay wrote in his landmark book *Achilles in Vietnam: Trauma and the Undoing of Character:*

> We must create our own new models of heal-
> ing which emphasize communalization of the
> trauma. Combat veterans and American citizenry
> should meet together face to face in daylight, and
> listen, and watch and weep, just as citizen-soldiers
> did in the theater at the foot of the Acropolis. We
> need a modern equivalent of Athenian tragedy.

In my own way, with the performance of Sophocles's
Ajax and *Philoctetes* for Marines in San Diego, then for
mixed military-civilian audiences across the country
and the world, I was hoping to answer Shay's challenge
to create a vehicle that would help Americans to come
together to share the burden of the pollution of war.

The archeological record suggests that every spring
at the Theater of Dionysus, the audience was seated according to tribe, which was, as Shay has pointed out,
according to military unit, and according to rank. The
only women to be present for these dramatic performances would likely have been the high priestesses, who
sat in the front row, alongside the general officers, in

appointed thrones that were inscribed with their names and titles.

Before the performance began that night in San Diego, I scanned the crowd congregating in the Hyatt Ballroom, with its harsh fluorescent lighting and worn wall-to-wall carpeting. I noticed Marines in clusters, which I presumed were units (or tribes). Young Marines gravitated toward the back of the ballroom and older, more seasoned ones congregated closer to the front. Though there were women in attendance that night, the majority of the audience was male, which should come as no surprise, since the Corps is roughly 94 percent male. Finally, I saw a cluster of middle-aged women, in relatively formal attire, move with near-perfect posture down the middle aisle, single file, and sit in the front row before what looked to be paper nameplates.

One of the women caught my eye and made a bee-line for where I was standing on the makeshift stage, a raised platform at the base of the ballroom. She reached up, took my hand, looked deeply into my eyes, and said with an unsettling blend of formality and familiarity, "Hi, Bryan. I'm Bonnie." I soon learned that she was the wife of the second most powerful general in the Marine Corps.

"It's lovely to meet you, Bonnie," I replied. "We're thrilled to be here." I quickly introduced her to the actors, who nodded respectfully in her direction. After an appropriate amount of time passed, I attempted to retrieve my hand from Bonnie's.

But she grasped it tightly, leaned in closer, and said, with suspicion and conviction: "I *know* you are here to perform an act of love." She continued to hold my hand, as well as my gaze, as if to leave no doubt in my mind as to the subtext of her statement: *You had better be here to perform an act of love.*

"We are," I said with confidence. Then, fearing she was far from convinced, I smiled and repeated myself: "We *are.*"

She slowly released my hand from her power grip and returned to her seat in the front row, flanked by the other generals' wives, the "high priestesses" of the Hyatt Regency. (I have since learned that the wives of Marine Corps generals hold a special place of prominence in their communities, one that affords them power and stature that is not always extended to the spouses of generals in the other services.)

Then the performance began. Vocal cords were shredded. Spit flew. And the actors fully committed themselves to the extreme emotions and anguish in Sophocles's words. Women throughout the room wiped tears from their faces as Ajax's wife, Tecmessa, put words to their worst fears:

TECMESSA
How can I say
something
that should never
be spoken?

You would
rather
die

than hear
what I'm
about to say.

A divine madness
poisoned his mind,
tainting his name
during the night.

Our home is
a slaughterhouse,
littered with cow
carcasses and
goats gushing
thick blood, throats
slit, horn-to-horn,
by his hand,
evil omens
of things to come.

Marines shifted in their seats with discomfort, as
Ajax called out for the deaths, not just of the gener-
als who had betrayed him, but of every warrior in the
Greek army:

AJAX
I call upon the Furies,
those long-striding
dread maidens who
avenge humans and

see to their endless
suffering: witness
how the generals
have destroyed me!

Train your eyes on
those evil men,
snatch them with
your talons and,
just as I die at
my own hands,
may they also be
murdered by their
own flesh and blood.

It's feeding time!

Gorge yourselves
on the generals
and their men,
fiercely descend
upon the army,
devour it whole,
spare no soldier!

Minutes later many audience members covered
their ears, as the warrior Philoctetes wailed in agony
as the mysterious disease ravaged his broken body,
calling out for death to visit him and release him from
the pain.

PHILOCTETES
Ahhhhhhhhhhhhhhhhh!
I have a sinking feeling,
your prayer will not
be honored by the gods,
for as we speak, blood
is oozing from the sore,
a dark red sign of evil
things to come. The pain
swells underneath my foot.
I feel it moving upward,
tightening my chest.
OH I AM WRETCHED!
Don't go. Please. Don't go.
You understand. You know.
Ahhhhhhhhh. Stay with me.
I wish they could feel this,
Odysseus and the generals.
DEATH! DEATH! DEATH!
Where are you? Why, after
all these years of calling,
have you not appeared?

When the performance ended, it was followed by a long, powerful silence. Then came overwhelming applause—a standing ovation that lasted several minutes. The plays had clearly struck a nerve. But it was unclear what would happen next—if people would be willing to speak, and what they would say.

To help break the ice for the discussion, I had

worked with the conference planners to identify three members of the community—a spouse, a Marine, and a psychiatrist—to form a panel to respond to the plays, in the moment, from their guts. They were to talk about what they had heard and seen in the plays that resonated with their own experiences, at war and while caring for those who had been to war. These panel members would serve the role of the ancient Greek chorus, intermediaries between the plays and the audience. I hoped they would model the kind of candid, heartfelt responses I wished to elicit from the Marines themselves. I had asked the panelists to come without prepared remarks or any special foreknowledge of the plays, and to respond sincerely to the lines that touched them most deeply and rang true to them across time.

One panelist, a beautiful, perfectly kempt woman in her mid-forties, with blond hair, striking blue eyes, and an unassuming voice, leaned into her table mike, looked out at the audience, and said:

"Hello, my name is Marshele Waddell. I am the proud mother of a Marine and the wife of a Navy SEAL. My husband went away four times to war, and each time he returned, like Ajax, dragging invisible bodies into our house. The war came home with him. And to quote from the play, 'Our home is a slaughterhouse.'"

The Marines all held their breath. In the back, a small group congregated around the cash bar, nursing Budweisers, gazing at the floor and waiting out the silence.

Marshele continued with her emotionally charged remarks. She quoted lines spoken by Tecmessa in desperation as she tried to persuade Ajax's men to help her save her husband: "How can I say something that should never be spoken? You would rather die than hear what I'm about to say."

And for a moment, the body language in the room suggested that Marshele might be right. She was speaking the truth of her experiences as a caregiver and as a military spouse, and as painful as it was to say and to hear, she was also opening a space for other spouses in the room to speak their personal truths.

The panelists finished their brief opening remarks and received a strong, supportive round of applause. I thanked them for their candor and bravery and turned to face the audience.

"Now is the time when we'd like to hear from you," I said. "Were there lines of dialogue or moments in the plays that spoke to you or resonated with your experiences at war, returning from war, or caring for those who've been to war?"

I gestured toward the microphones, on stands, that had been placed at the front and rear of the center aisle, and waited to see if anyone would stand up and speak. After a long, awkward silence, much to my disappointment, a few people stood up and offered predictable, rote statements about how we should support veterans and place our faith in God. This was followed by a heavier, seemingly interminable silence.

Finally, a short nun, who I later learned was a chaplain in the Canadian army, approached the microphone with a small piece of paper in her hands. She adjusted the microphone, stretching it down to her face, and then stood silently for several seconds, pregnant with speech, clearly debating whether to say what was on her mind.

Then she lifted up her head to read carefully and deliberately from her notes: "I would like to repeat a line from the play *Ajax* that I have heard countless young men say to me over decades of serving alongside them in multiple wars: 'Witness how the generals have destroyed me!'"

Bonnie, the assistant commandant's wife, shot up in the front row, not even bothering to approach the mike, and shouted something to the following effect: "How dare you say that! Our husbands made this conference possible. This is about healing, not assigning blame!"

The crowd recoiled at the unfolding conflict between the nun and the general's wife.

Just when it seemed that things couldn't get any worse, Marshele jumped into the fray and spoke directly to Bonnie, who was still fuming at the front of the ballroom: "I can definitely relate to that line, too. Over the years, my husband has said things like that to me. He's felt that way on many occasions."

By this point, the tension in the room had risen to such a boil that I was scanning for the nearest exit, in case we needed to make a quick getaway.

Marshele's remark prompted a second general's wife to stand up and go on the attack, accusing her and the nun of purposely undermining their husbands' authority.

Marshele responded calmly, without sounding the

least bit defensive. "I did not mean to say anything disrespectful about your husband, ma'am. I am simply repeating something that my husband, who is a Navy SEAL, not a Marine, has said in the past."

And before I knew it, at least thirty people had lined up to speak at the microphones. Each person, whether he or she responded directly to the nun or to the generals' wives or to Marshele—leadership was just one of many themes that emerged during the discussion—quoted lines from *Ajax* and *Philoctetes*, without consulting notes, as if they had known Sophocles's plays their entire lives. They interwove their comments about the plays with their own experiences with such prosody and rhetoric that it seemed Sophocles himself had written their monologues.

The event reached its dramatic climax when a charismatic African American sergeant major stood up and delivered, full tilt, a sermon about the price of leadership, aiming his words in the direction of the generals' wives in the front row. "To be a leader means that ninety-nine percent of the time you try to do the right thing, but it doesn't mean, just because you're a leader, that you always end up doing the right thing."

A large portion of the diverse audience called to him: "You say it, brother!"

"To be a leader means that your decisions are going to cost lives, and so even if you do the right thing, there are families of Marines who you will have lost in battle, who will never think you did the right thing, no matter what you say."

"Amen."

The sergeant major had emerged as the chorus leader, bridging the world of the play with the world of the audience. At times, it wasn't clear whether he was quoting from the play or speaking extemporaneously, so impassioned and dramatically compelling was his speech. He was taking a huge risk speaking publicly to the generals' wives in this manner, but his delivery was so eloquent and powerful that he rallied the rest of the audience to stand behind him and chant its support in unison. I later learned that he received a phone call from Marine Corps headquarters in Quantico, Virginia, that night, inquiring about what he had said, but that in the end he was not disciplined.

We had scheduled forty-five minutes for the audience discussion, but it continued well into the night. After more than three hours, I had to cut it off, but it clearly could have lasted until dawn.

The next morning, as the actors and I were preparing to leave the hotel for the airport, an AP reporter who had been assigned to cover the event walked over to me and asked with sly amusement, "You do realize that there were three generals sitting in the back row last night?"

I stopped in my tracks, wide-eyed at the revelation. Clearly everyone else in the audience had been fully aware of it. The discussion, I saw, had been conducted in such a way that no one had addressed generals directly—the closest they had come was through their wives. Everyone had been speaking to the generals and to each other in a highly coded manner that I had barely apprehended.

Standing in the Hyatt lobby, I realized something about the power of ancient Greek drama, both in the ancient world and today, that I could not have known until I heard four hundred Marines and their spouses responding to Sophocles's words. Thanks to the U.S. Marine Corps, we had peered into the ancient past and had come into contact with an aspect of the performance that I believe—though I have no way of proving it—must have been taking place within the confines of the Theater of Dionysus during the fifth century BC.

I saw firsthand that these ancient plays possess the power to disrupt rigid hierarchies, at least temporarily, and to give warriors of all ranks permission to bear witness to the truth of the experience of war. Tragedy was not simply a matter of entertainment. It was an ancient technology. That night in San Diego, plugged into the right audience, Sophocles's plays had done what they were designed to do.

III

On May 11, 2009, Sergeant John Russell walked into the Combat Stress Clinic at Camp Liberty, Iraq, a massive military complex near the Baghdad airport, sat down in front of the psychiatrist on duty, and reportedly declared, "You are either going to help me, or I am going to kill myself." Less than an hour later an army doctor, a navy social worker, and three soldiers lay dead on the clinic floor.

At the time of the killings, Sergeant Russell, age forty-four, was on his fifth deployment to a combat zone—including Bosnia and Kosovo—since he had first enlisted in the Army National Guard in 1988. But according to his mother, Beth Russell, who testified before a military judge during an investigative hearing, his nightmares didn't begin until just before his third deployment to Iraq, in 2008. It was then that she noticed him losing sleep and eating less, and she became concerned.

In the days leading up to the attack, Sergeant Russell's fellow soldiers had noted changes in his behavior. He had become detached, lethargic at work, and overly suspicious that the members of his unit were conspiring to end his career and send him home for good.

After Sergeant Russell confided to a staff sergeant that the situation in the unit "made him feel like he wanted to kill somebody," he was brought to see a chaplain, who recommended that he seek professional help. On May 8, he visited the Camp Stryker Stress Clinic in search of assistance.

In 2009, for a noncommissioned officer in the army to pursue mental health treatment in such a public way, in a combat zone, would have been a potentially career-killing act, given the long-standing, heavily entrenched stigma associated with mental illness in the U.S. military. Conversations with mental health professionals are not deemed confidential, as they are, by law, in the

civilian world. Everything that Sergeant Russell dis-
closed in the clinic could, and most likely would, immediately be reported to his command. To this day, many
service members still see psychological injury, or combat stress, as a character flaw or sign of weakness.

According to the testimony of one psychiatric nurse,
the army psychologist on duty treated Sergeant Russell sternly. As the nurse observed with discomfort, the
major interrogated him for nearly twenty-five minutes.
"I experienced it as being aggressive and hostile," the
nurse remembered, "and I know Sergeant Russell felt
very uncomfortable, and he kept looking for reassur-
ance, but what do you do when a senior officer is there?
You don't do anything; you sit, and you listen."

Instead of being immediately treated for severe depression "with psychotic features" and "chronic post-
traumatic stress disorder," as a medical panel from
Walter Reed Army Medical Center later diagnosed his
condition, Sergeant Russell was reprimanded and referred to the Camp Liberty Combat Stress Clinic.
There he met with a clinical social worker who apparently joked around during their session, minimizing his
troubles, then referred him to an army psychiatrist for
treatment. According to his defense attorney, Sergeant
Russell felt he had been openly mocked at the clinic.
He felt doubly betrayed, by the medical staff and by his
unit, and he was consequently even more reluctant to
return for help. After leaving the Camp Liberty clinic,
he was so visibly rattled that a lieutenant from his unit,
upon observing him, took away the bolt from his rifle.

On May 10, Sergeant Russell was brought back to the Camp Liberty clinic to meet with an army psychiatrist, who diagnosed him as having an "anxiety disorder" and prescribed an antidepressant. He was to return to the clinic in a week for another visit, but in the hours that followed, his mental state rapidly deteriorated. Soldiers from his unit observed him weeping and trembling. Others heard him stuttering and talking about hurting himself. He was coming apart.

The next day Sergeant Russell was escorted to the Camp Liberty clinic for acute care, and it was then that he reportedly issued his ultimatum to an army psychiatrist—help me, or I will end my life. Whatever took place next—the details are not clear—he left the clinic and then returned moments later with a weapon, which he used to gun down the social worker who had mocked him, as well as an army doctor and three enlisted soldiers.

Article 90 of the Uniform Code of Military Justice prohibits any service member from assaulting a superior officer. Any service member who "strikes his superior commissioned officer or draws up or lifts up any weapon or offers any violence against him while he is in the execution of his office" is subject to punishment—including death, if the offense takes place during the conduct of war. In 2012 a military judge determined that Sergeant Russell was fit to stand trial and would be judged in accordance with the law, in spite of his mental

illness. In May 2013 he was found guilty of premedi-
tated murder and sentenced to life in prison without
parole.

Although the Camp Liberty clinic shooting was one
of the most gruesome acts of soldier-on-soldier violence
in the Iraq War, the story of Sergeant John Russell isn't
unique. It has been repeated countless times throughout the world, for as long as humans have waged war. It
is a story of invisible wounds, perceived betrayal, military "justice," and the true cost of war. It is a story that
could have been taken right out of the pages of Sophocles's *Ajax*.

In the prologue to *Ajax,* the goddess Athena appears
on account of two violations of military justice, one by
Ajax and the other by Odysseus. Under cover of night,
Ajax has lifted his weapon against superior officers,
after being passed over for the honor of receiving the
armor of the slain Achilles. His fellow officer, Odysseus, has arrived at Ajax's camp at dawn, pursuing an
"enemy."

Athena punishes both men for these violations. Just
before Ajax attempts to strike his so-called enemies—
Agamemnon, Menelaus, and Odysseus—she blinds
him with divine madness and sends him reeling into a
field full of animals, where, in a berserk rage, he slaughters and tortures cows, goats, and sheep, believing them
to be the very men he came to kill.

Then in turn, she exposes Odysseus, against his will,
to Ajax's mental illness, admonishing him never "to say
an arrogant word against the gods again, or stick out

your chest because of your strength or your abundant wealth. In just one day, all things living can be lifted up, then buried deep below." By the end of the scene, Odysseus, humbled and awestruck by the destruction of the mightiest of all Greek warriors by an invisible sickness, lays down his weapon and says to Athena, "I feel sorry for him, though he hates me. I see now that we are nothing but insubstantial shadows."

In the Theater of Dionysus, when *Ajax* was first performed,* the significance of this scene could not have been lost upon the thousands of war-torn citizen-soldiers who watched this ancient drama play out, on the stage and in their lives. The general officer and playwright, Sophocles, was speaking to them through Athena, goddess of wisdom and war, about the core values and fundamental tenets of military justice.

By depicting the "divine madness" inflicted upon Ajax by Athena, Sophocles was also speaking of the psychological damage of war. He was not the only ancient author to write about combat trauma. As Jonathan Shay has pointed out, Homer's *Iliad* and *Odyssey* read like catalogs of combat trauma and psychological wounds—most notably the poisonous effects of betrayal, guilt, exhaustion, and grief upon warriors, during and after military conflict. The narrative structure

---

* The dating of Sophocles's *Ajax* is unclear. Many scholars consider it to be one of his early plays and place it in the 450s or 440s. Some tragedies of the fifth century BC were performed again in fourth- and third-century revivals. *Ajax* is known to have received multiple restagings during the centuries that followed its premiere.

of the *Odyssey* hinges upon a scene in Book 8 in which Odysseus, on his way home from Troy, is waylaid on the opulent island of Phaeacia. There at a banquet he hears a bard sing about the Trojan War. The songs, recounting stories of fallen friends, trigger Odysseus emotionally, causing him to break down in front of his hosts and tell them the story of his long journey home.

The fifth-century Greek historian Herodotus recounts a story of an Athenian soldier, Epizelus, who in the thick of the Battle of Marathon in 490 BC suddenly goes blind, "though he had not been struck or hit on any part of his body. But from this time on and for the rest of his life, he continued to be blind." And in perhaps the most gruesome depiction of combat trauma and its aftereffects to survive the ancient world, Euripides's play *Madness of Heracles* includes a horrifying scene in which the Greek hero and combat veteran Heracles goes on a killing spree in his own home, executing his wife and children—at least one point-blank with his weapon—mistaking them for his enemies.

Little is known about how performances of ancient Greek tragedies affected audiences in fifth-century Athens. What little source material exists suggests that the Greeks were not passive observers. Aristotle describes lively, raucous crowds who would whistle performers offstage if they didn't like the performances. And one apocryphal legend, recounted in an unreliable biography of Aeschylus that was written during the Alexandrian period, depicts an incident at the premiere of his *Eumenides* in 458 BC. When the savage Furies—horrifying birdlike goddesses of vengeance—first took the stage to stalk the matricidal murderer Orestes, apparently the audience was so petrified by the sight that "children fainted and unborn infants were aborted."

This last account, while most likely untrue, illustrates how later generations viewed the potential impact of Greek tragedy upon audiences. As I have already argued, any tragedy worth the price of admission, in fifth-century Athens or today, does something to us—physically, spiritually, biochemically. It shocks us. It rearranges our molecules. Appallingly violent scenes like the suicide of Ajax or the massacre in Euripides's *Madness of Heracles,* I would argue, were not staged for their entertainment value. They were staged in order to elicit a specific response from a specific audience.

Scholars have often referred to Sophocles's *Ajax* as a "problem play." Though the date of the text is unclear, some see it as the flawed work of a young dramatist, suffering from an overly simplistic plot structure and dramatic inertia. Others are baffled by the fact that the protagonist dies halfway through the story and his body remains on stage during the final acts, as officers in the Greek army argue about whether to give it a proper burial. For these reasons and more, *Ajax* has often been passed over by professors and stage directors alike in favor of Sophocles's traditionally better-regarded plays—*Oedipus the King* and *Antigone.* This historic preference dates back over two thousand years to Aristotle's *Poetics,* which holds up *Oedipus the King* as one of the finest examples of Greek tragedy while critiquing *Ajax* for its simple plot structure; that negative judgment has unwittingly trickled down to the modern reader. Consequently, very few people have ever read or seen *Ajax*.

While the plot of *Ajax* arguably does not progress with the rich complexity of *Oedipus the King,* in recent years the play has revealed itself to be far more insightful and textured than originally thought. As it turns out, Sophocles had something profound and timeless to say about the experience of war, something that an educated readership largely untouched by military conflict has all too frequently overlooked and undervalued.

At the center of the tragedy is the suicide of a combat veteran, one of the most graphic and iconic depictions of suicide in all of Western literature. Sophocles staged the violence of Ajax's death mere feet from where the generals* sat in the audience in the ancient Theater of Dionysus. But he did something else equally remarkable: he cleared the *skene,* or "stage," of all other characters and took the audience inside the mind of a person who is actively contemplating suicide, deep inside the insidious logic that leads him to end his own life.

---

* Since the dating of *Ajax* is unclear, it is impossible to know if Sophocles was serving as a general at the time the play premiered. It is believed that Sophocles was first elected general during the suppression of the revolt on Samos (441–439 BC), which maps to the possible dating of *Ajax* to the late 440s BC, favored by some scholars.

During the wars in Iraq and Afghanistan, the rate of suicide among active-duty U.S. service members sky-rocketed. The U.S. military has made great efforts to reduce the stigma associated with seeking help for mental illness and suicidal feelings, but the number of suicides among active-duty service members remains high.

Most of these suicides take place within the lower enlisted ranks, though generals and admirals have taken their own lives, too. Startlingly, a study in the *Journal of the American Medical Association Psychiatry* found that between 2004 and 2009 the suicide rate for soldiers who served in Iraq and Afghanistan doubled, but the suicide rate among service members who never deployed to the battlefront tripled. Moreover, most of the enlisted service members with suicidal tendencies had first experienced them before they enlisted. These findings complicate an already mysterious phenomenon, but Sophocles's *Ajax* may shed light on the underlying reasons behind some military suicides.

While the play describes the unraveling of a combat veteran, the trigger that sets him off is related not to combat but to the internal politics of the Greek army. *Ajax* kills himself for many reasons, including grief, shame, exhaustion, anger, and guilt. But it is the feeling that those above him in the chain of command have devalued and betrayed him, both as a warrior and as a man, that ultimately sends him to his death. One needn't go to war to feel devalued or betrayed. It can happen anywhere, especially in a society that does not value the sacrifices of its warrior class.

Billions of dollars have been spent trying to devise effective interventions that will stem the rising tide of suicide in the military, but researchers have barely begun to scratch the surface of the issue. The science is new, and very little is known about who will ultimately commit suicide or how to tell that someone is contemplating it. By depicting the innermost thoughts of an ancient warrior who is in the throes of suicidal thoughts, thereby humanizing his ambivalence and articulating his despair, Sophocles's *Ajax* provides a clear perspective on the internal struggles of service members and veterans today.

In the play, a few short moments before Ajax takes his own life on a sand dune by the sea, he prays to the Olympian gods for a "quick and easy death."

> AJAX
> I call out to Hermes,
> escort of the dead,
> who delivers men
> to the underworld,
> to guide this sword
> as it pierces my rib-
> cage so it skewers
> my heart and ends
> my life instantly,
> sparing me pain
> after the plunge.

He prays to the Sun, to deliver the news of his death to his family back home:

I call out to you, Helios,
as your burning chariot
streaks across the sky,
when you come to my
home, pull back your
blazing reins and pause
to announce my death
to my poor old father
and to the pitiful woman
who nursed me as a child.

Then, overwhelmed with emotion, the hardened warrior breaks down in tears:

No doubt, when she hears
the news, her wailing will
be heard through the hills.

But he immediately shuts down his feelings, stuffing them back inside:

No more talk of tears.
It's time.

Death oh Death,
come now and
visit me.

Then, just before throwing his body upon the blade of Hector's sword, he hesitates—ever so briefly—and voices his internal struggle:

But I shall miss
the light of day
and the sacred
fields of Salamis,
where I played as
a boy, and great
Athens, and all
my friends.

In these penultimate lines, we hear Ajax's ambivalence about whether to live or to die. Even at this moment, the decision to take his own life is not a foregone conclusion. As he remembers the people and places that have made his life worth living, he wrestles with what to do. Then, searching for the fortitude and the energy to follow through with his plan, he calls out to the "springs and rivers, fields and plains" that "nourished" him while at Troy, to witness his death.

These are the last
words you will
hear Ajax speak.

He impales himself on his sword and gasps for air.

The rest I shall say
to those who listen
in the world below.

After one performance of *Ajax* at a U.S. Army installation, a soldier stood up and said, "I knew Ajax was thinking about killing himself when he deceived his family and troops, and walked away from his tent brandishing a weapon. But I don't think Ajax *knew* he was going to kill himself until he was alone on the sand dune with his gods." At a later performance on an air force base, a pilot shouted out, "Those were his demons!" I think the operative word is *alone*. In how many ways, intentionally and unintentionally, do we leave soldiers like Ajax alone to do battle with their darkest thoughts and memories? *Ajax* challenges us to sit uncomfortably with this question, as we watch a decorated soldier come apart before our eyes.

In 2010, while I was in Athens to give a talk, I visited the Theater of Dionysus at sunset and—while no one was looking—slipped into one of the thrones down front, in which the ancient generals once sat. I stretched out my feet and imagined what it must have been like to see Ajax—alone on stage before an audience of thousands—voice his most private thoughts of rage, ambivalence, and despair before taking his life a short distance from where I was sitting. The play seemed to ask a crucial question: *At what cost?*

For centuries, Westerners have struggled to find words to describe the psychological impact of war upon those who wage it. During the American Civil War, combat veterans displaying the symptoms of mental illness and other related stress reactions were diagnosed with *soldier's heart* or *exhausted heart*. In 1905 the Russian army coined the term *battle shock;* Russia was the first major country to classify combat-related mental illness as a legitimate medical condition. With the advent of high-caliber weapons during World War I, the phrase *shell shock* was coined in an attempt to forge a direct link between the emotional turbulence of war and the concussive injuries inflicted by heavy artillery. The term *combat fatigue* was also used widely at that time. During World War II, the phrase *thousand-yard stare,* inspired by the vacant, emotionless gaze of war-torn veterans, was introduced to the mainstream American vernacular. Finally, in clinical settings during World War II, the medical term *gross stress reaction* began to be used as a crude diagnosis for the invisible wounds of war.

For decades, and throughout subsequent conflicts such as the Vietnam War, many of these now-antiquated phrases remained in common circulation as the clinical understanding of war-related psychological injury and how best to treat it progressed at a glacial pace. Then in 1980, the diagnosis post-traumatic stress disorder, or PTSD, was added by the American Psychiatric Association to the third edition of its *Diagnostic and Statistical Manual of Mental Disorders* (DSM III), in effect reducing all previous attempts to describe the psychological impact of war to a sterile, scientific-sounding acronym.

Critics of the term *PTSD,* including military mental health professionals, are many and vocal: they feel that labeling the condition a "disorder" pathologizes people who are experiencing a normal reaction to abnormal circumstances—such as the trauma of war, sexual assault, or a natural disaster. Also, all too often, a wide range of temporary and nondebilitating reactions to stress are lumped under the diagnosis, further stigmatizing the full spectrum of responses to war that most veterans experience. In other words, not every veteran who has nightmares or who jumps whenever a car backfires has PTSD. But in the popular imagination, the larger societal stigma associated with mental illness and the stereotypes perpetuated by films and television leave little room for this distinction.

Jonathan Shay describes PTSD as "the persistence into civilian life, after danger, of the valid adaptations you made to stay alive when other people were trying to kill you." He too has been openly critical of the term and the way it has been used in recent years as a catch-all. He refers to PTSD and its attendant symptoms as the "primary injury," but has argued that many veterans are suffering from something far more insidious, destructive, and complex than the neurological symptoms resulting from exposure to war-related trauma. Rather, it is something of a spiritual and moral nature that he and a growing number of prominent mental health professionals now refer to as *moral injury*.

Though not a formal diagnosis and still widely controversial, the concept of moral injury continues to gain momentum in clinical settings, even within the military. At its core, moral injury is about betrayal and primarily, according to Shay, "betrayal of 'what's right' in a high-stakes situation by someone who holds power." Betrayal, he and his colleagues argue, cuts in many directions. A warrior can feel betrayed when a higher-ranking officer orders him to do something wrong. Or perhaps more subtly, a warrior's sense of right and wrong can be turned on its head when he witnesses or feels complicit in something that goes against his moral compass. A warrior can betray himself when, in the heat of battle, he makes a split-second decision that results in the death of innocents, soldiers, or friends. And a warrior, like Ajax or Sergeant Russell, who perceives that he has been betrayed can end up betraying his family and friends, and his fellow warriors, by committing an act of violence or taking his own life.

In recent decades, as asymmetrical, counter-insurgency-based warfare has proliferated—ever blurring the lines between enemy and civilian, battlefield and neighborhood—the potential for such betrayals seems to have proliferated as well. Moral injury may, in fact, be the signature wound of the wars in Iraq and Afghanistan, not only during deployments but also when veterans return from war to pink slips, skyrocketing unemployment, and an apathetic, disengaged nation. Betrayal might just be the wound that cuts the deepest.

When I first started presenting Greek tragedies to combat veterans, mental health professionals expressed two pervasive knee-jerk concerns: (1) the performances would "retraumatize" veterans with PTSD, activating their symptoms and sending them into a tailspin of anxiety, depression, and suicidal thoughts; and (2) the plays, hitherto the province solely of academics and the elite, would fly straight over the heads of those in the lower enlisted ranks, many of whom had never been to college and likely never encountered ancient Greece outside comic books, video games such as *God of War,* and films like *300* and *Troy.* Sure, the plays had moved a roomful of Marines in San Diego, but were they really appropriate for infantry? Sophocles's tragedies were incredibly violent—depicting massacres and a suicide on stage—and featured aggrieved warriors expressing unbridled rage: rage at fellow soldiers, rage at their command. Would performing them on a military installation be constructive? Or would it simply fan the flames, inciting the very emotions being expressed on stage?

In order to gain access to "boots on the ground" soldiers and find out whether the plays spoke to them, I would need to convince the gatekeepers of the army to let us perform on bases. So I spent the first year of the project showcasing *Ajax* and *Philoctetes* for military doctors and psychiatrists, as well as for generals and high-level Department of Defense officials. After an early performance for just such an audience in Maryland, a trained sniper/medic—a killer and a healer—remarked that the play was a more realistic depiction of war than any television show or movie he had ever seen. When I asked why, he replied, "The violence of war is swift and decisive. The violence of Ajax was swift and decisive." If he had experienced something palpable and real about war in the play, something that transcended time, then other combat veterans, regardless of rank, would surely experience it, too.

I was glad that he spoke first that day, for his brief

remarks seemed to validate what had happened in the Hyatt ballroom in San Diego. Those who had gone to war and come into contact with death, who put their lives on the line, who had lost friends and soldiered on and who knew the meaning of sacrifice, had no trouble understanding Sophocles's plays, regardless of their level of education or exposure to the Greeks.

Perhaps more than any other extant Greek tragedy, Sophocles's *Ajax* has at its center an act of violence so unthinkably gruesome that over the course of the play it is described three times, with increasing urgency and detail. It's almost as if the play itself is post-traumatic, repeating the story again and again in a frantic attempt to make sense of the violence, or to temper its effects with language. Ajax may not have been a wordsmith, but he knew how to express himself with a sword—conveying all his pent-up rage, shame, and grief through a grammar of blood and entrails. Violence was a language that many in Sophocles's audience, like the sniper/medic in Maryland, intrinsically understood.

Sometime in the fifth century BC, when the play premiered in the Theater of Dionysus, the violence of Ajax must have unlocked something buried deep within the men in attendance, something that transcended language—a scream. Ancient Greek contains many sounds that function as words, and the name *Ajax* (or *Aias*) is one of them. Etymologically, it is the sound of a blood-curdling scream, a cry of anguish and despair. And in Sophocles's version of the story, Ajax realizes the true meaning of his name in the final hour of his life, while howling in suicidal despair:

AJAX
Ajax.
Ajax.

My name is a sad song.

Who would
have thought
it would some-
day become
the sound a man
makes in despair?
Ajax.

In the late winter of 2009, after a series of success-
ful pilot performances for military audiences, I found
myself sitting in the Arlington, Virginia, office of U.S.
Army brigadier general Loree Sutton. Her imposing desert boots propped against the far edge of a conference
table, she leaned back in her chair and rattled off her
vision for my project, rapid fire, to a group of colonels
and their support staff. She pointed her finger around
the room like a gun. "Here's what we do, gang. We
rent football stadiums. Pack them with soldiers—thirty
thousand a performance."

Earlier that fall I had traveled to Washington, D.C.,
with a group of actors to perform scenes from Sophocles's plays at a Department of Defense conference on
"Warrior Resilience." It was at that conference that I
met General Sutton. One of her staff members, Lieu-

tenant Colonel Mary Hull, had attended our Marine
Corps performance in August and brought word of the
project's early success back to her office. Upon Hull's
recommendation, the conference planners had inserted
our program—now branded Theater of War—into the
lunch hour.

During the performance that day, before a crowd
of 250 military leaders, some of them with two and
three stars on their lapels, the actor Paul Giamatti bel-
lowed the bone-chilling invectives of the abandoned
veteran Philoctetes as he rages against the nation that
has betrayed him and left him to die on the island of
Lemnos. After it was over, a heavy silence pervaded the
room.

General Sutton stood up, her hands visibly trembling, and addressed her peers. "Perhaps Sophocles
wrote these plays," she said, "because he was in the
minority as a leader with regard to the compassion he
felt for the warriors in his community who were struggling with the issues he portrayed in his plays. Perhaps,"
she concluded, "Sophocles wrote these plays to comfort
the afflicted and afflict the comfortable."

I knew we had struck a chord. At the time, General
Sutton was the highest-ranking mental health professional in the U.S. military, and the first female psychiatrist to rise to the rank of flag officer. In the fallout of
the Walter Reed scandal, Congress had appropriated
hundreds of millions of dollars to address the mental
health needs of returning veterans, and General Sutton
had been tasked by the Department of Defense with the

enormous responsibility of leading the effort to heal the invisible wounds of war. This meant increasing the number of psychological resources available on military installations all over the world. It also meant identifying and supporting novel approaches to eliminating the stigma associated with soldiers seeking help.

From the outset, the scale of the problem before her was vast and daunting, which explained why, when I met with her in her Arlington office, she led with the idea of staging Sophocles's plays for thirty thousand soldiers. "Time is not our friend," she said repeatedly during that first meeting.

I struggled to convince her that although Sophocles's original audience could have easily filled half a football stadium, the scale of Theater of War performances would need to be much smaller in order to create a safe, intimate environment for soldiers to speak openly and without fear of retribution.

But the demand was so great, and the issues so immense, she replied, that we could spend the rest of our lives presenting Sophocles's plays to U.S. military audiences and reach just a small fraction of those who had served in Iraq and Afghanistan. "Never," she said, "has so great a burden been placed on the shoulders of so few on behalf of so many for so long."

The discussions about the scale and scope of the proposed tour lasted nearly a year. After a grueling governmental contracting process, we finally reached a compromise—one hundred performances over a twelve-month period on military installations throughout the world. We would target 200 to 500 service members per performance, and we would leverage national media to reach millions more. At least, that was the plan when I embarked upon an unprecedented partnership with the U.S. military to resurrect an ancient general and bring his healing message to thousands who needed to hear it.

AMERICAN AJAX

I

Ajax could no longer remember the man he had been
before the war. Though nine years had passed since
he first came to Troy, it might as well have been ninety.
With each fighting season, the conflict had spread,
almost imperceptibly, back into his perception of the
past, infecting his earliest childhood memories. Nothing remained untainted. Now it consumed his future, or
what little he had left. Soon he would be dead. By the
time death came for him, he wouldn't mind.

He'd seen enough, more than most men see and do
in ten lifetimes. Some mornings, before predawn raids,
he would think about his three-year-old son, or his
aging mother back home waiting for the slightest sign
of his return, and weep behind his shield, so the soldiers
wouldn't sense his weakness. "Crying is for women and
for cowards," he told them over and over again. "The
only time I cry is at funerals."

The only man with whom he had shared his grief was
Achilles. Early in the war they had been sitting together,

rolling a die, playing a game, passing the time between campaigns. Suddenly, without warning, he found himself balled up in the dirt, sobbing. Then, as quickly as it had come on, it was over. He picked himself up and dusted himself off. They shared a look. And that was all he needed.

Now that Achilles was dead, taken down by the enemy (with the help of a god) in the ninth year of the war, he had no one to share in his sorrow. Certainly not his half-brother, Teucer, who would immediately take away his weapon and relieve him of his command. And certainly not his wife, Tecmessa, who would never understand. Even if he wanted to tell her, he lacked the words. He'd never been good with words. The only language he really knew was violence.

When Achilles died, no one mourned his loss more than Ajax. And yet Ajax kept his sorrow close, carrying it deep within his chest. His father, Telamon, a decorated war hero, had raised him never to show his emotions. All he knew to do was suck it up and soldier on with the fight.

They called Ajax "the shield" because he shielded the army from the worst of attacks. He and his unit were always the farthest downrange, fighting in forward locations, laying their lives on the line and sustaining the greatest losses. As a leader, it had been his job to protect his men. And the burden of survival now weighed more heavily on his shoulders than the body of his dead friend, which he carried slowly, mournfully, over his shoulder, off the battlefield.

To call it survivor's guilt does little justice to what it's like to lose a friend this way. It's more than guilt. It is an overwhelming sense of failure, as well as a mystery. "Why am I here when he is not?" Ajax asked himself as he trudged back to the camp with Achilles on his back. "This isn't how it was supposed to be."

He'd witnessed the horrors of war—he'd seen innocent children die, soldiers cut to pieces, and ravenous fires consume whole villages alive, burning them to ashes. But nothing affected him more than the death of Achilles. He trudged back to his tent on the outskirts of the encampment and tried to avoid the prying eyes of his wife all night. He couldn't so much as glance in the direction of his son, whom he loved more than life itself, without feeling his knees start to buckle.

The next day, when he reported for duty, the commanding generals, Agamemnon and Menelaus, gathered the troops for an announcement. Morale was understandably at an all-time low, they said, after the death of Achilles. And so they would suspend all operations and hold three days of funeral games, to celebrate the life of the greatest Greek warrior before he was laid to rest. There would be competitions of strength and endurance. Whoever emerged the all-around victor would win the grand prize of Achilles's armor, which everyone knew was the greatest honor one could receive in the Trojan War.

Ajax glared at Agamemnon as he spoke with sudden, newfound respect for Achilles, which he had utterly lacked while Achilles was alive. War was political—this much he knew. But he wanted no part of the politics. Would Agamemnon speak of him this way after he was gone? The thought nauseated him, as did the idea of playing games over armor that everyone knew should rightfully go to him. Achilles had been the greatest warrior in the army—this was undisputed. But Ajax was the strongest. He was also Achilles's cousin.

Over the first two days of the funeral games, Ajax effortlessly bested all his fellow warriors in the contests of strength and endurance. No one came close to his scores. But on the third day, he stepped into an arena in which he lacked the skills to compete: each of the top contenders was to make a speech about why he deserved the armor of Achilles. They were provided no time to prepare and could not consult notes. They would have twenty minutes.

After drawing lots, Ajax was to go third. Except for giving orders to his men and screaming at new recruits, he had never delivered a public speech before. He was a man of action, not of words. And so when it came time for him to speak, he found that he could not summon a sentence, nor will his mouth to move. After a long, awkward, seemingly interminable silence, he finally managed to utter three words: "I am Ajax." Then he thought better of saying anything more. The statement alone should stand for itself, he thought. What more could be said?

No one dared laugh as Ajax held the judges' gaze. They would wait until he was well out of earshot before bursting into uproarious laughter. But what happened then was no laughing matter.

The next contender, Odysseus, approached the crowd with tears welling in his eyes. "My fellow warriors," he began his speech, "I wish I had the words to express my sorrow at losing such a great and noble friend."

Odysseus had been called "the man of many turns" because he contradicted himself so often, flip-flopping his position on any issue if he saw the potential for political gain. In many ways, he had been the architect of the war—the director of Greek intelligence. Behind closed doors, from the safety of the camps, he had made decisions that had won battles but had also cost the lives of those who fought in the trenches. Odysseus represented a new breed of warrior, one who saw honor in deceiving his enemy, as well as his friends, as long as it meant winning in the end.

Odysseus delivered a beautiful, perfectly structured speech about how Achilles had been his closest friend, in whom he had confided his darkest fears and secret griefs. His loss would be felt for generations to come. The speech was filled with duplicity and lies, yet in delivering it Odysseus did the soldiers a great service, providing them with a rare opportunity to grieve. For by the time his twenty minutes were up, every man in the audience had wept into his hands until he ran out of tears—except Ajax.

When the judges declared Odysseus the overall winner and presented him with Achilles's armor, Ajax showed no emotion. He turned away from the crowd, from his own men, who stood stunned and awaiting his orders, and walked back to his tent, his face as unreadable as stone.

The first official Theater of War tour stop sponsored by the Department of Defense (DOD) took place on October 16, 2009, in a restored nineteenth-century opera house in Junction City, Kansas. The audience included roughly 150 infantry soldiers from the Second Brigade of the army's storied First Infantry Division, otherwise known as "the Big Red One"—famous for sending the first American troops into battle in all major conflicts over the last hundred years, from World War I to the wars in Iraq and Afghanistan. The soldiers had returned from Iraq to nearby Fort Riley only ten days before.

Colonel Kevin Brown, the garrison commander, was a charming young leader with an earnest but hardened all-American demeanor. During a prior rotation at Fort Drum, New York, he had encountered a soldier who had become a modern-day Ajax. The soldier had returned from a challenging deployment to Iraq with the Tenth Mountain Division, in which he had lost several good friends. Shortly after his return, his wife had left him. The soldier had then tied up his wife's dogs and savagely beat them to death.

When he learned about the soldier's actions, Colonel Brown felt an overwhelming sense of helplessness and horror as he imagined the chain of events that had led him to vent his frustration and grief upon defenseless animals. Sometime later he had read about Theater of War in *The Atlantic Monthly*. He hadn't been casually reading the magazine—he had been scouring the Internet for solutions, desperate to find a way of reaching the soldiers under his command before they became Ajax. Once he realized what we were doing, he had fought for us to come to his installation first. He wanted to expose his soldiers, along with their spouses, to Sophocles's plays, as a way of helping them reintegrate back into their domestic lives.

Under Colonel Brown's direction, the support staff at Fort Riley pulled out all the stops, organizing a reception for the soldiers when they arrived, handing out pamphlets and specially made "command coins" with a suicide hotline number engraved on the back, making sure that every seat in the opera house was filled with a soldier, spouse, or mental health professional. Major General Vincent Brooks, an elegant African American second-generation general, gave the introductory remarks, asking the soldiers "to open yourselves up to the performance, to really take it in." ("Theater," he would later tell me after a performance at an army base in Kuwait, fifteen miles south of the Iraq border, "is the best medium for conveying the spirit of something.") He asked the soldiers to stand and be applauded for their service.

Then, in a startling act of leadership, he asked all the mental health professionals to do the same. This was the first time in the Fort Riley community that soldiers and counselors had been brought together to engage in open dialogue, and General Brooks, it seemed, intended to set the tone by establishing that everyone was standing on even ground. The general then took his seat next to his wife in one of the gilded boxes and, sitting ramrod straight, observed the event from above the crowd.

The reading of scenes from Sophocles's plays that night was especially powerful, featuring explosive, gut-wrenching performances by the actors Adam Driver, Joanne Tucker, Jay O. Sanders, and Michael Stuhlbarg. Inspired both by the setting and the audience, they left nothing on the table.

One audience member, Major Jeff Hall, leaned forward to watch Ajax rage against his superiors and descend into depression and madness. Major Hall had deployed twice to Iraq and had returned from his most recent deployment physically injured and psychologically broken. I had first met Jeff and his wife, Sheri, at an army health conference in New Mexico, where we had been showcasing Theater of War in the summer of 2009. They had been flown there from Fort Riley, Kansas, by the Deployment Health Clinical Center at Walter Reed to serve as panelists. Jeff later said that during that first encounter with Sophocles's plays he had thought, "My God, that's exactly how I feel. That's exactly how I acted. And it dawned on me that this has been something, an issue, that's been going on for twenty-five hundred years, and the Greeks, this is the way they dealt with it. They would bring in their regiments to watch these things so they could cope."

Promptly after the performance in Junction City, a panel of community members replaced the actors on stage, including a chaplain, a psychiatrist, and Jeff and Sheri Hall, who since the New Mexico performance the previous summer had become evangelists for Theater of War. All of them told heartbreaking, captivating stories, but it was the Halls who broke things open that night. While Jeff sat stone-faced on stage, Sheri spoke haltingly, tears streaming down her face, occasionally pausing to clear her throat or blow her nose.

"Hi, my name is Sheri. When my husband, Jeff, came back from Iraq the second time, I looked into his eyes, and I didn't recognize the man I had married nearly twenty years ago. We had been high school sweethearts, but it was like looking at a stranger. His eyes were as black as night and filled with hatred, not for me or for our girls, but for people in his own command who had betrayed him.

"Things hit rock bottom when I found Jeff out in the front yard one night with an empty bottle, cradling his pistol. He had that stare that Ajax's wife, Tecmessa, talked about. He said he didn't want to live anymore. I asked him to think about me, about the girls, and what his death would do to our family. . . ." By the end of her remarks, there wasn't a dry eye in the auditorium.

Then, as the audience settled into their seats to begin sharing stories, Colonel Brown addressed the crowd again, compelled to speak, to name something that for centuries had been customarily swept under the rug. "These plays were written long ago," he said, pacing the lip of the stage with manic intensity, "but they describe people I know." He pulled out a newspaper article from a camouflaged pocket, the one about the soldier at Fort Drum, and read it aloud like a script.

Meeting Colonel Brown and getting to know the Halls and their two lovely girls, Courtney and Tami, affirmed all my hopes for Theater of War and what it aimed to achieve. The Halls, in many ways, were a living testament to the enduring power of Greek tragedy. By recognizing themselves in the actions and behaviors of Ajax and Tecmessa, they seemed to gain much-needed perspective—a longer view, so to speak, of their own private struggles. The more they shared and the more I listened, the clearer it became that the story of Ajax was their story. It was a story they needed to tell, over and over, until it somehow made sense. The story belonged to them.

In those early days, people would compliment me on "coming up with the concept" behind the project. But I soon began to understand that the project was having a profound influence on me as well, shaping my character and the course of my life in ways that I could never have anticipated when I first sat down to translate Sophocles's words. I suddenly felt an overwhelming sense of responsibility, as the privileged guest in a world that few civilians had been allowed to visit, and as the keeper of stories that had never before been spoken.

During those early months of the tour, as I listened to the responses of audiences throughout the country, I realized that the Halls were not alone. To them and to thousands of other military families, Sophocles's plays were not museum pieces or "problem plays," as classicists had so often labeled them; nor were the performances jarringly extreme. To them, no matter how abrasive or emotionally charged the actors' voices became, this was kitchen-sink realism.

11

When I interviewed Jeff Hall for this book, he told me unequivocally that he had fallen in love with the army as a young boy. If you asked his mother, he said, she'd tell you that he'd joined when he was five years old. All the men in his family, including his father and uncles and the men they worked with, had served during times of war—World War II, Korea, and Vietnam. Jeff remembers growing up in the Oklahoma panhandle and hearing stories about all the "grandiose, awesome, dreamland stuff that military people do." Listening to their war stories, he saw his destiny stretch out before him like the seemingly endless plains and prairies.

He met Sheri in high school, when he was a sophomore and she was a junior. She still tells people that she "married her stalker," because he used to follow her around town after school and never talked to her, never said a word. He seemed quiet and shy, according to Sheri, and she "kinda fell in love with him from the beginning." When prom season came around, it was she who approached him, on a dare. He said yes.

Early in their dating, he told her that he planned to join the army and warned her there was nothing she could do to change his mind. At first, she felt like he was trying to preemptively break up with her, but she was secretly impressed by his drive and determination. He said to her, "If you stick with me, we'll go places." And they did.

When he was seventeen, Jeff turned down several

college football scholarships and enlisted in the army two weeks after his high school graduation. He shipped off to basic training in the summer of 1988 to become a heavy-wheel vehicle mechanic. For as long as he could remember, he had wanted to be an infantryman and fight on the front lines. But his father, whose memories of the Vietnam War were still fresh, made him promise that he'd choose a specialty that would keep him from the front lines.

Jeff and Sheri were married by a justice of the peace on January 1, 1991, while he was home from Germany on fifteen days' leave. Technically a war bride—the Gulf War had begun the previous August—she braced herself for Jeff's inevitable deployment to Iraq, but two months later the war came to an end. She moved to Germany and stayed there with him until he left the army later that year and enrolled in the ROTC program at Emporia State University in Kansas. "The second he signed those discharge papers, he knew he'd made a mistake," she remembers. "I could just tell." Within a year of leaving the army, he would be trying to find a way back, any way he could.

Upon Jeff's graduation from college, the army commissioned him as an officer in the field artillery branch. His first assignment was to Fort Wainwright, Alaska, with the 411th Field Artillery, where he trained in light infantry and fire support. During that time, he traveled all over the world, to Japan, Guam, and Kenya. "I was living the dream," he recalled. "I was light infantryman. Plus I was a fire support officer. I loved it. I was at home with that. I like everything forward. And that's always been my taste. I've always wanted to be on the cutting edge of where everything was." He had finally found his way to the front lines.

While he began to realize his childhood dream, he and Sheri brought two beautiful children into the world, less than two years apart, Tami and Courtney. And, as with all military families, Sheri and the girls followed Jeff wherever he was told to go, even to Alaska. Sheri didn't mind the separation from her own family. She knew that traveling was part of the itinerant life of an army wife. In a way, when her husband first joined the army, she had enlisted alongside him. Inevitably, she knew, there would be separation and isolation. But the Halls vowed that their military life would bring them together as a family and draw them closer. They decided to "make [their] own memories."

The girls adjusted well to military life, and Sheri loved the social aspects of being an officer's wife. She made fast friends and fit in well with the other wives. It was a very exciting time, even while Jeff was deployed to Guam. The Halls were stationed in Alaska from 1998 to 2001, when they returned to Fort Sill, Oklahoma, where Jeff was ordered to take the Captains Career Course.

Everything for this young military couple seemed to be moving along according to plan. Sheri remembers thinking of Jeff, "What a wonderful, amazing person this is who wants to serve his country. He wanted to be a war fighter." And she kept thinking, "We'll never go to war again, and if we do, it will only last a hundred hours." But then on the morning of September 11, 2001, two planes hit the twin towers in lower Manhattan, and instantly everything changed. Sheri saw Jeff go immediately into what she calls "battle mode."

He woke up that morning, turned on the *Today* show, and "watched the breaking news that one of the towers had been hit." He called his mother and watched the second airplane hit the south tower. "We're under attack," he told her. According to Sheri, he immediately said: "I'm ready to go right now. Forget the training. I need to get as quickly as possible with any unit that's headed over there. I need to go now."

The Halls waited an excruciating six months before he was assigned a duty station, where he would even have a possibility of deployment. "The way we fight today," he remembers thinking, "the war will be over before I get out of here. Man, I'm going to miss it again." In June 2002 the Halls were sent to Fort Riley, Kansas, and within weeks of arriving, they received word that Jeff's unit would be deploying to Iraq as early as January 2003.

Jeff and his unit spent the next few months training to go to war. All the while, Sheri stood on the sidelines, just as she had since high school, and provided unconditional support. "That was my job, as a military spouse, as a mother, as a wife. I had to support what he did, because what he did was going to keep us all alive and free. That may be a fairy tale to some people, but that's how I saw him. He was going to be our saving hero." In April 2003 she and the girls said goodbye to Jeff, fighting back tears, trying to remain strong.

Soon after Jeff arrived in Baghdad, his battalion commander approached him about becoming the leader of
a motorized rifle unit called the COLT platoon. Jeff
jumped at the opportunity and immediately began putting together a plan to transform the platoon into the
"primary raid and quick-reaction force for the battalion." It ensured that he and his soldiers would always be
on the front lines, where all the action would be.

Jeff describes himself as a "kid in a candy store"
in combat. He had trained all his life to fight, to put
his life on the line, to defeat the enemy through overwhelming force. "When we were going out and kicking
that ass, I had no issues whatsoever. But it was when
we started getting our ass kicked, and we wouldn't do
anything about it, that it started to affect me." For his
entire career, he had been trained to "gain and maintain
superior firepower over your enemy, maneuver close,
and kill"—a lesson, he said, he and his fellow soldiers
learned "in blood." He believed in the effectiveness of
force and aggression to preserve American lives. Once
you established dominance in a firefight, he said, the
enemy left you alone. "If you want to go home," he
repeated, "you will be the aggressor."

But in Iraq, he would discover that Operation Iraqi
Freedom was a much different war from the ones
he had trained for, at least in terms of the way it was
being fought. The rules of engagement had changed.
He remembers discovering this one night early in his
first deployment, when a man on a rooftop began fir-

ing rounds down upon two of his vehicles, riddling their roofs with bullets. Jeff and his soldiers immediately returned fire, spraying fourteen hundred rounds in the shooter's direction, killing him and demonstrating what might become of anyone else contemplating doing the same. According to Jeff, they "did everything we were trained to do." But when he called his battalion commander to request permission to break contact and return to the forward operating base, his commander replied, "You will go back and guard the body," and "I need the Social Security number of every person who fired their weapon."

A minute ago, thought Jeff, the shooter had been "trying to kill us," and now he and his soldiers were the ones "on trial." In a matter of seconds, his world had been turned upside down. He suddenly found himself fighting in a war that the army, he felt, was not trying to win. "We don't even know what winning is," he concluded. In order to bring his soldiers home safely—as he had vowed to do—he would now have to protect them from his superiors and their strategies.

A few hours later Jeff discovered that the colonel who had ordered him and his soldiers to stand by the body of the man who had just tried to kill them, placing them unnecessarily in harm's way, was stationed at a commandeered mansion—called the Pool House—on the outskirts of the city, completely disconnected from the dangers of downtown Baghdad. The commander's distance from the fight, coupled with his disregard for the soldiers' safety, engendered a sense of resentment in Jeff that would fester in the months ahead.

Jeff and his COLT platoon continued to do what they had been trained to do. They volunteered to go on perilous raids, knocked down doors, got shot at, returned fire, and searched for high-level people who were on the run. They even caught one of Saddam Hussein's bodyguards, about a week before the Iraqi leader himself was captured. In spite of the command environment and the orders coming from above, Jeff tried to maintain his platoon's aggressiveness, all the while asking himself, *What is the end state? What are we trying to do here?*

The first improvised explosive device, or IED—of the six that would eventually fragment his memories and rattle his brain—detonated in between two of his vehicles. Neither vehicle was armored. Though the device was relatively small, the blast was enough to blow the windows out of the second vehicle, and Jeff's driver "looked like Freddy Krueger after that, literally. His face was just eaten off with shrapnel and gravel from the road."

That IED was another turning point in Jeff's experience of the war, not on account of the blast itself but because all along the road, Iraqis stood cheering. "They were starting to believe that we were just occupiers," he recalled. "We were risking our lives for these damn people, and they didn't seem to care. They were cheering because I had a wounded guy on the road. And how I kept my guys from shooting them, I don't know, but we didn't shoot anybody." Pausing, he remarked, "In some ways it still haunts my dreams that we didn't do it. We sucked it up and drove on, like we always do."

Jeff rarely spoke to Sheri during his first deployment. He wanted to keep the two worlds separate—the home front and battlefront—and thought that by cutting off communication, he could better focus on the task at hand: getting his soldiers home alive. But in August his battalion commander walked up, handed him a satellite phone, and said, "Call your wife." He reluctantly followed orders, dialing Sheri's cell.

They talked for about ten minutes, mostly about their daughters and quotidian things back home. Then he paused and said, "We've lost this war." And when Sheri asked why, he replied, "We've changed all our language. We have stopped being aggressive, and now we're starting to get hurt." Something about saying out loud what he had been thinking made his thoughts harder to silence. "It was kind of the tipping point for me," he remembered.

Then the battalion lost its first soldier—killed in action—when shrapnel from a roadside IED ripped through the canvas door of his vehicle, striking him in the head. "I remember him being stripped naked by the medics," Jeff said, "because they couldn't find where he had been wounded and they were frantically trying to find the wound. Eventually, they found a small hole just above what would have been his left ear." The medics tried their best to keep the soldier alive until he could be medevacked to a field hospital. When the chopper came in, they were still working on him, as the dust blew in plumes, swirling around them. Jeff grabbed the soldier's face and cradled it against his chest, so the sand would stay out of his eyes, but the chopper couldn't land and, when it lifted back up into the air, Jeff saw sand in the soldier's eyes. They were gray.

And Jeff thought, *Oh my god, this kid is dead. He's nineteen years old. My god, this kid is dead.* He looked around at his soldiers. "And I'd never seen these looks on their faces, 'cause this was the first time they'd experienced death to one of our guys. And they looked like 'Oh my God, we are not bulletproof.' And, of course, I launched right into drill sergeant mode and got everybody moving and up, got everyone back on that horse and told them to ride. And I remember being affected by this kid's death, but not in the manner that I thought I would be. I thought that maybe I would cry some, but I didn't. I just went right back to work. Right back to work."

Shortly after their first soldier was KIA, or killed in action, the battalion "chalked up" two more fatalities. But by then Jeff and his soldiers were starting to get used to the constant threat of death and the reality that any day could be their last. There would be many more casualties in the months ahead. Each time it happened, their job would be to not let it affect them. Their job would be to go back to work.

III

Technically, Tecmessa wasn't Ajax's wife. She was his battle-bride, and theirs was a marriage born from trauma. Ajax had slaughtered her brothers, as well as her father, when he raided their home in Phrygia—set it all ablaze. Every once in a while, it would catch up with her, the weight of what had happened, but then she would shrug it off as nostalgia for a world that no longer existed.

She loved Ajax out of necessity. Without him, she and her son would be slaves. With him, they were a family. In time, she truly came to love him. And as she got to know him—the real him—she found plenty to love. It didn't hurt that he was handsome, courageous, selfless, and kind—at least, behind closed doors. He wasn't always generous to his men, but that was for their own good. She could no longer remember life before he liberated her from Phrygia, before he took her hand by force.

During her time in Ajax's tent, she had grown accustomed to the incidents. Countless times over the years she had awakened, gasping for breath, as her husband's hands closed tightly around her throat. Those had become routine—they came with the territory of being a warrior's wife. At first she had pleaded for her life, but she quickly resorted to biting, scratching, and clawing away at his broad chest, while stifling the impulse to scream, for fear of waking the baby. Then when he came to his senses, she'd hold him close and console him for losing control and mistaking her for the enemy.

Or there were the less dramatic but no less shameful events. They would be sitting down for a meal, and suddenly his eyes would recede into bottomless pools of black. She would wave her hand in front of his face and snap her fingers, but no one was home. And she'd know by looking at him, slumped forward in his chair and staring into the distance, sometimes for seconds, sometimes for hours, his head tilted slightly toward the floor. When he returned, he'd never remember having left. They would go about their lives as if nothing had happened.

Of late, these absences occurred with greater frequency. Every time, when it was over, she thought about asking where he had been but then thought better of it. The one time she tried to speak of it, he cut her off and said, "Woman, silence becomes a woman." She'd heard him say that before, and she knew what it meant, so she left it alone and prayed for the war to end soon.

Tecmessa was a minor character in Greek mythology, a Phrygian princess whose only real claim to fame was that Ajax the Great conquered her land and took her as his war prize. Yet Sophocles purposefully placed her at the center of his play, gave her a comparable number of lines to his central character, bestowed her with Ajax's young son, and assigned her some of the most moving speeches in the entire play. In ancient times the role of

Tecmessa would have been performed by a male actor for what was likely a mostly male audience. Though strong female characters in Greek tragedy—such as Clytemnestra, Medea, Antigone, Hecuba, and Electra—were in no short supply, it does seem significant that Sophocles chose to foreground the struggles of an army wife in front of an audience comprised of male soldiers. By setting the main action of the play in front of the tent on the outskirts of Troy, where Ajax lived with his battle-bride and their three-year-old son, Sophocles—in effect—brought the home front to the battlefront, shining a spotlight upon the collateral damage incurred by military families during times of war.

In the play, after he awakens from his blind rage, Ajax finds himself lying upon a mound of slaughtered carcasses, and he discovers that he has "stained his hands with the blood of cows." He vows—in front of his wife and his troops—to "do something bold" that will "erase all doubt" in his father's mind that he is "anything but a coward." In no uncertain terms, he begins talking about taking his own life.

Tecmessa summons all the strength she has left. She gets right in Ajax's face and jabs and swings at him until she finds an exposed nerve, hoping to jar him loose from the insidious logic of his suicidal thoughts. In an effort to bring this scene to life for military audiences, some of the actresses who have played Tecmessa have resorted at this moment to physically striking the actor playing Ajax, slapping his face and beating his chest, hoping to somehow penetrate his defenses and touch his heart:

TECMESSA
Think about your father, whom you
will be abandoning in the throes of
old age, and your poor old mother,
who spends all her days praying that
you will some day return home alive.

And what about your son?

Can you imagine how hard
your death will be on him,
growing up fatherless and
without food on the table,
living with men who hate
him for being your son?

I have nowhere else to go,
no one to whom I can turn.

My parents are dead.
You destroyed my
homeland. You now
are my homeland,
my safety, my life.

Nothing else matters but you!

I ask you to remember
all the good times
we had and to treat

me kindly, for a noble
man always remembers
those who gave him
pleasure and protects
them from danger.

Sheri had prepared herself for little to no contact
during Jeff's first deployment. On the day he left, she
said to him, "Call me when you get to Kuwait, if you
can, and call me when you get back to Kuwait, and
when you're on your way home." She thought it would
be reassuring for him to hear her say that. But that year
it took all her strength, strength she didn't know she
had, to hold the family together. In her mind, that was
her job. She had to be strong. She held on to the belief
that Jeff and his soldiers were well trained, and that
things would be okay.

But when news came back to Kansas of the battalion's first KIA—the young specialist—and then, one
week later, the death of a captain, suddenly the war
became real, and the thought of death began to invade
and colonize her consciousness. She lived with constant
awareness that Jeff and his soldiers were in mortal danger, and she spent her nights praying that she "wouldn't
get a knock at the door one day."

On the day Jeff returned from his first thirteen-
month deployment to Iraq, Sheri and the girls were
beside themselves with anticipation. "To describe a
redeployment ceremony, it's a lot of anxiety, 'cause you
haven't seen this person in a year. I have never seen the

kids so excited. Not even on Christmas morning." It was Easter Sunday. Patriotic music was blaring, reverberating through the cavernous hangar in which the families of the 4-1 Field Artillery, Third Brigade, First Armored Division were waiting to see their soldiers. A general was addressing the crowd. Jeff's parents and sister were standing by their side. *Honestly,* Sheri recalled thinking, *if this general doesn't quit speaking, I'm going to be the one on the national news when I jump over these chairs and run out there.* It was the longest ten minutes of her life.

The first thing he said, after embracing her and the girls, was "I just want to go home." Minutes earlier, before dismissing the soldiers from formation, the commanding general had informed them that they would all be returning to Iraq in twelve months, which meant, in practical terms, that Jeff would be flying out again in ten. Of those, he would be home for three—that is, when he wasn't training. Later that night Jeff broke the news to Sheri, and soon thereafter they told the girls, who didn't take it very well but understood that it was "part of the deal" when your dad is in the army. Sheri remembers making a conscious decision to "stay in deployment mode." As a family, they never let down their guard; nor did they ever get used to Jeff being home. So by the time he finally returned from his second deployment, they would have been at war for more than three years.

When Jeff came back from his first tour, he had looked and acted very much like the man Sheri had known since high school. He had been sobered by war and was no longer idealistic about the mission, but he remained motivated and engaged and was driven to work harder, to give more of himself to his job, by a strengthened sense of obligation to protect his soldiers from both the army and the enemy.

But when he returned from his second tour, two days after Christmas 2005, Sheri knew immediately, even seeing him in the hangar, that something was different. He ripped off his Kevlar and tossed his helmet onto the ground faster than before, grabbed his girls, and held them close. "I saw a lost soul," she remembered. "I saw a shell of a man. His eyes didn't light up. He was there, but he wasn't there. And I could tell. I could *tell*. He had just a deep dark look. It was like looking into two black holes. And I just knew deep down inside that something wasn't right and this was probably going to be the start of a very long road for us." Something had happened this time around.

The girls unwrapped the presents still waiting under the tree, having patiently deferred Christmas until after their father's return, and went to bed. Then Sheri gently approached Jeff and said, "Something is wrong. I can tell by looking at you," to which he dismissively replied, "I'm fine. I'll be okay." But she pressed on. "If you need to go talk to somebody, you need to go talk to somebody. Don't keep it in." But that's where their conversation ended.

Army counselors assured Jeff that it was normal to be angry and that his sensitivity to things would eventually subside. So Sheri and Jeff resolved to sweep it all under the rug, soldier on, and hope things would get better. For a while, according to Sheri, they struggled to "fake it," at least for the sake of outward appearances. But Jeff's anger began to flare uncontrollably, without warning, and things quickly got real.

That July they moved to Fort Polk, Louisiana, where he had been assigned to work as an instructor at the Joint Readiness Training Center, preparing the next generation of soldiers for the grueling ground battles that awaited them in Iraq and Afghanistan. They sold their Kansas house, and during a two-week transition, while living in a motel, Sheri remembers Jeff becoming enraged when Courtney, their younger daughter, audibly complained—whining and rolling her eyes—when Jeff asked her to retrieve something from the car. He "turned red and his eyes got black," Sheri said. "And the three of us are sitting on the bed in a Motel Six, and we're listening to him and he's pointing his fingers and Courtney's crying, practically hiding behind me. She's crying, and Tami's just looking at him like 'Who the hell are you?'"

He went into the bathroom and slammed the door. A few minutes later he came out and said, "Um, I'm going to go out for a while," and left. Sheri turned to her sobbing daughter and said, "The next time your dad asks you to do something, just do it! For godsakes, just do it."

It was the first time he had taken his rage out on the girls, but not the first time he'd shown it to Sheri. On several occasions since he'd come home he had unloaded his anger on her, calling her names, then five minutes later forgetting all the hateful things he had said. It was as if he were someone else during the rants. It was like watching explosions detonate inside his mind, obliterating all trace of what had set them off.

When they arrived at Fort Polk, Sheri again suggested to Jeff that he "talk to somebody." His response was the same: "I'll be fine." The pattern continued, on and off, for the next two and a half years. One day he would be fine, acting like himself, and another day he would be filled with rage, which only seemed exacerbated by work. Sheri remembers him coming home and shouting in frustration that the army was lying to young soldiers about the type of war they would be fighting and then sending them over—poorly trained—to Iraq to get killed.

When the surge came, and the operational tempo shifted toward punishing back-to-back deployments, with no family time and just a week off between rotations, Jeff increasingly felt complicit in perpetuating the lie, as well as helpless to protect his trainees from the army that was mobilizing them in unprecedented numbers to fight for unheard-of durations. Daily reports came back to Fort Polk listing the soldiers who had died. Jeff didn't want to see any of the soldiers he had trained on the list, so he worked harder and harder in the hope of saving lives.

He committed himself to his job with the same drive and focus with which he approached his deployments, silencing thoughts of his home life when he was on the job. He began working around the clock, shutting everything and everyone out. "All the family time, all the great things we had thought we were going to do in Louisiana, went out the window," Sheri said. "Forget it. Didn't happen."

Then Jeff started isolating himself in more obvious ways, avoiding his wife and children. Again, Sheri suggested that he go see someone. This time he did, a psychiatrist who prescribed three bottles of pills, which Jeff quickly tossed aside. The last thing he wanted to be was "medicated."

"We stopped talking to each other. I stopped asking. He stopped telling me," Sheri said. On a particular morning in April 2008, she was driving the girls to school, when Courtney turned to her and said, "Dad said he thinks he's having a midlife crisis." Sheri paused and thought, *Why is my thirteen-year-old daughter telling me about this?* Then she replied, "I think Daddy's just having a hard time. Work's got him down. He's mad at work. I think he'll be okay." She dropped off the girls and headed back to the house.

She found Jeff still home, getting ready to leave. They both stood in the kitchen, waiting through a long, awkward silence. Then Sheri blurted, "Courtney said you think you're having a midlife crisis."

Jeff sat down and rested his head on the kitchen table. "I don't know what's wrong with me," he moaned.

"Well, I think you might need to go talk to somebody different and try to find out what's wrong with you," she countered. "You're sick of wearing this uniform. You're sick of working with soldiers. And if you're done with this family, with this marriage, you need to tell me right now. I can't help you if you don't want me to."

Jeff stood up and without another word went to work, just as he had done before, but when he came home that night, something was visibly different about the way he carried himself. All life had left him. He seemed defeated. The next morning he woke up and said, "I don't want to go to work. I can't go to work. I can't put my uniform on." That—as Sheri remembered it—was the beginning of his descent into the darkest depression.

He wanted to be alone. He told her to take the kids and leave. "I just want to die. If I die, everything will be better," he said over and over again.

It got to the point where she was afraid to leave him at the house when she went to run an errand or pick up the girls from school. She stopped eating and sleeping and dropped a lot of weight. "I would lie in bed at night," she said, "watching him sleep, because I was scared that he would get up and take that pistol that was in the drawer, with the loaded clip in it, and go somewhere." Whenever she and the girls arrived home from school, Sheri would race into the house to make sure Jeff was sitting at his computer or in a chair, and they weren't coming home to brains on the wall and a corpse. "I did not want them to come home and find that," Sheri said.

One night, shortly after Sheri dozed off into fitful sleep, she awoke to an empty bed. She frantically searched the house but saw no sign of her husband. Then she heard a noise in the front yard. She swung open the door and spotted him, out in the middle of the lawn, gesturing wildly. He'd consumed three bottles of homemade wine and was having an animated conversation with their dog. From where she was standing, it looked like he was responding to things the dog was saying, as if the dog had been talking back to him.

She helped him inside, then scooped up the bottles from the lawn and somehow managed to get him into bed. When he awoke, she asked him what he remembered from the night before. He remembered talking to the dog. More unsettling, he remembered the dog talking back. Also, he remembered carrying a loaded weapon—the clip was in the gun—and talking with the dog about whether to pull the trigger.

She looked him straight in the eye. "I cleaned up your mess in the yard last night so the kids wouldn't see it," she said. "But I'll be damned if I'm going to clean your brains off the bedroom wall. *You have got to get help!* You have got to find out why you feel this way. If you kill yourself, how will I explain it to your daughters, your parents, your sisters, your entire family?"

"Everybody will be better off without me," he replied.

"Nobody's going to be better off without you," she shot back. "You are the only one who's going to be better if you're not here. You're the one who's not going to have pain anymore. I'll have to live with that for the rest of my life. Your kids are going to have unanswered questions forever."

He fell silent. Something about what she said had landed. His thoughts were swirling in a new direction. He opened his mouth and quietly muttered, "I don't want my kids to find me in the yard with a bullet hole in my head," almost ashamed to say the words. He told her he would get help.

But she was skeptical. She'd heard him say that before. "Honestly, I didn't think we'd be together much longer. Either he'd pack up and leave, or he'd kill himself. 'Cause I wasn't leaving. I was never going to leave."

IV

When Jeff and Sheri Hall first heard about Theater of War and were invited to participate in the community panel at the army health conference in New Mexico, they went out and bought a copy of Sophocles's *Ajax* at the local bookstore. One page into reading it, she turned to him and said, "This is the part of English literature that I hated in high school. I'm sorry. You read it." He flipped quickly through a few more pages, glanced up at Sheri, and said, "We're just going to have to wing it."

When the reading began, and the performers started ripping into the material, screaming and wailing with anguish and desperation, the Halls' mouths fell open in astonishment.

The actor playing Ajax turned red, the veins in his

neck bulging, his eyes bottomless black holes, and began screaming at Tecmessa, "Will you not leave me alone? Will you not go?" Jeff and Sheri's eyes met. "That was you," she whispered in his ear, to which he replied, "That is me. That *is* me."

And when Sheri heard the actress playing Tecmessa plead with her husband to think about the impact his death would have on their family, Sheri thought:

That's me. I hid our kids away. I begged and pleaded for him to get help. And the only difference between her and me was I didn't go to his soldiers. Believe you me, I've taken hits from them for that. But I was embarrassed. I didn't want anyone to know that my hero was having a breakdown. But I said the same words. What can we do to fix this? I wanted to fix it. And when I think about the slaughtered animals, that was our family. Our children were innocent. They didn't do anything. And they were getting stepped on. And I was letting it happen in my own home. I let it happen. It was completely eye-opening. I was like, "Holy cow, people gotta know about this." And suddenly I wasn't embarrassed to tell my story anymore.

In the months that followed, Sheri and Jeff participated in the community panels for many Theater of War performances, including the one in Kansas and high-profile events in Washington, D.C., sometimes traveling great distances to tell their stories to audiences of strangers. Every time they spoke, their stories gained a little more clarity. Jeff, in particular, seemed to discover new things at every performance. It was stunning to watch him spontaneously sharing these fresh insights, just as they came to him, with audiences of soldiers and spouses.

The more he told his story, the better he seemed able to make sense of the events in Iraq that had precipitated his desire to die. The more he talked, relating his story to Sophocles's *Ajax,* the clearer it became that no single IED blast, or ambush, or soldier killed in action was to blame for his anger and depression. If anything, it was the cumulative impact of those two grinding deployments to Iraq that had slowly, insidiously pushed him over the edge.

Most tellingly, with each performance, he zeroed in on the moral dimensions of Ajax's madness. Ajax's rage, according to Jeff, sprang from his sense of having been betrayed. His world had been turned upside down by the corrupt behavior of his superiors, who by giving Achilles's armor to Odysseus had devalued his service and his sacrifice, taken away his identity, and stripped him of his ability to grieve. Their reckless decisions had obliterated his understanding of the world and his sense of justice. Blinded by grief and rage, Ajax betrayed himself. Consumed by shame, he took his own life, hoping it would extinguish the pain.

Fortunately, Jeff and Sheri, with the support of Jeff's command, found the help they needed—in an intensive three-week program at Walter Reed Army Medical Center—before it was too late. It helped the Halls begin talking to each other again. And interacting with other soldiers and spouses who were struggling with similar issues helped them put their problems in perspective and see that they weren't the only military couple desperately trying to hold it all together.

Though the impact of Sophocles's plays upon the Halls will never be quantified, recognizing themselves in the actions and words of Ajax and Tecmessa seemed to help ease their pain and put them on a path toward helping others. Through Theater of War, they began speaking out and sharing their stories, and the performances gave them permission to say things they had never spoken aloud, not even to each other in private. They began bringing Courtney and Tami to the events, so the girls could hear the truth of what the family had been through. On more than one occasion, I looked out into the audience while Jeff and Sheri were speaking and saw their daughters sobbing in their seats. The burden of that image was difficult to bear, perhaps more than any of the stories that the Halls told, for it was unclear to me whether the girls' presence at the events was healthy or helpful.

As we continued to tour military installations with the project, I often saw teenagers—the children of soldiers and Marines—sitting alongside their parents, listening attentively to the performances and to the adult themes of the town hall discussions. They seemed far from bored. In fact, from the way they took it all in, it appeared that they might share profound, unspoken insights into Sophocles's plays.

During one particularly challenging performance at the Army War College in Carlisle, Pennsylvania, as I struggled to get a roomful of colonels to begin talking openly about their reactions to *Ajax* and *Philoctetes,* I noticed a teenager, wearing a black jacket and tie, seated near the front of the auditorium next to his mother. As a rule, I try not to put anyone on the spot, but I could tell that he had something to say and drew him out:

"You, sir, look like you might have an answer to my question. Why do you think Sophocles wrote these plays? What was he trying to say or do?"

Without hesitating, the young man replied, "He wrote them to morally instruct his soldiers in what they should and should not do."

During a performance at Fort Drum, New York, a battalion commander talked about how he and his wife had tried to shelter their young daughter from death and from the horrors of war. But late one night, after the phone rang, the five-year-old came into their bedroom, rubbing her eyes, and asked, "Daddy, did a soldier die?"

The battalion commander scooped up his daughter and said, "What makes you ask that, darling?"

"Every time the phone rings late at night, it means another soldier died," she said. The battalion commander suddenly understood that there was no way to shelter his daughter from war, and that she intuitively comprehended more about death than he had imagined possible.

In one variant of the myth surrounding the death of Ajax, his three-year-old son, Eurysaces, goes on to become a great king. I have often marveled at how that might have happened, how a child who grew up in a war zone—surrounded by death and destruction—and who lost his father to suicide, could grow up to become a functional adult, let alone the king of Salamis. But the more time I have spent with military children, the better I have come to understand their unique strength and resilience, forged by a relentlessly itinerant existence and by an early understanding of death and of the mortal danger of their parents' profession.

Years later Courtney Hall, Jeff and Sheri's younger daughter, shared with me that nothing that her parents had spoken on stage came as a surprise to her or her sister, yet she felt that the performances had been a positive force in their lives. They had brought the darkness that had enshrouded her childhood out into the light. They had eliminated the shame and the silence that surrounds mental health issues in military culture. They had given her parents a language for talking about something for which they previously had few words. And they had helped others follow her parents' example. Theater of War, she said, had saved her family.

In the year that followed our first official performance of the DOD-sponsored tour, in the Junction City opera house, I spent nearly three weeks of every month on the road. We performed for infantry Marines, Navy SEALs, drone pilots, fighter pilots, generals, privates, soldiers, military families living at home and abroad, and even the airmen and -women who preside over our nuclear arsenal. Everywhere we traveled, we heard the most powerful, revealing, insightful things said about Sophocles's plays by individuals and communities who had lived the experiences they portray. The more we toured, the more humbling it was to see—night after night—that the audience always understood more than we did about Greek tragedy.

Not all the stories people told were of trauma or loss. Many recounted tales of inner strength, recovery, and resilience. Some of the most inspiring stories were about loyalty, fidelity, and acts of selflessness and kindness that reaffirmed, night after night, my faith in humanity. A majority of the people who spoke had been made stronger by their war-related experiences and expressed a deep appreciation for life and its fragility. Hearing their stories filled me with an inexplicable optimism, which fueled my resolve to continue performing, sometimes more than five times a week.

Six months after our appearance at Junction City, we were invited back to Fort Riley to present a special performance for spouses whose loved ones were deployed to the Middle East. We presented an entirely new cut of *Ajax,* which did not end with the suicide scene but continued through to the end of Sophocles's tragedy, depicting the impact of the suicide upon Ajax's wife, son, and troops, as well as the entire chain of command.

The panel that night consisted of five spouses, in-

cluding one woman who had lost her husband to suicide. After the performance, the widow—slowly and
methodically—recounted the story of her husband returning from a deployment to Iraq. Within weeks, he
had become so paranoid and debilitated by fear that he
could barely leave their bedroom. He came mentally un-
glued. In the days leading up to his death, he could no
longer distinguish between horrifying flashbacks and
reality. Most important, he could no longer distinguish
between the enemy at his doorstep and his family. He
discovered himself—in one lucid moment—planning to
kill his wife and children and at that moment decided to
take his own life.

The widow told this harrowing story plainly, in a detached manner. She never cried or appeared to be fighting back emotions. She seemed practiced and numb.
All the other women on the panel sobbed uncontrollably through her story and their own. During the
panelists' remarks, at many moments, I heard guttural
noises coming from multiple locations in the darkened
audience.

In the front row, a stone-faced one-star general
named David Petersen sat beside his wife, taking it all
in. He had the thousand-yard stare. About halfway into
the audience discussion, a woman stood up in back
and directed her voice toward the widow on the panel.
"My husband came home from war and took his own
life. And it was just like your husband, ma'am. And
it was just like Ajax." For a moment, no one so much
as breathed. Toward the end of the evening, another

spouse stood up and—in her own words—said the same thing.

Afterward the stone-faced general approached me and said, "Well, that was . . . something," and walked away. And I thought to myself, *He clearly hated it. It cut too close to the bone. We'll never be able to return to this community again.*

But a few weeks later I received a phone call from a social worker at Walter Reed Army Medical Center, who said that the very same one-star general had flown to Washington, gathered a group of mental health professionals around a big table, and said: "I just saw this thing called Theater of War, and I need more resources for the families living in my community. People are hurting, and I felt helpless."

It was the first time we had clear confirmation the project had effected meaningful change at the leadership level. Later that year I asked General Petersen for a testimonial about his experience with Theater of War. Here's some of what he wrote:

> In the first place it is kind of hard to explain until it is actually experienced. The TOW I went to was designed for spouses. The play was read by well-known actors so was done very professionally. Following the play, which by itself is very powerful, we had a panel of five spouses who have lost their spouses due to suicide. That was followed by a facilitated discussion and comments from the audience. The stories we heard were hard to

listen to and very moving. The whole thing lasted for almost four hours, and we had to cut it off because it was a work night.

We had in the audience spouses, soldiers, and health care professionals as well as family and friends. It was one of the most uncomfortable and powerful things I have ever been involved in. I had a lump in my throat the whole time and was afraid I would shed a tear. That wouldn't have been a bad thing, but I was the senior person in attendance and sitting in the front row. I am not by nature a touchy-feely type guy, but it is very hard not to be involved.

The play is 2,500 years old and talks of suicide caused by the pressures of war and how different people deal with it. Since I have been here we have had nine soldier suicides and a number of dependents as well. This is my new family, and every loss hurts. We are looking at the TOW as a way for our soldiers and families to communicate and talk about issues to build resilience so they don't take that final step of taking their own life. . . .

We have had five showings here and are planning more. It's not magic, but it works if people are willing to open up and share experiences. We heard from spouses what it is like to be left at home dealing with all the everyday things of life as their soldier goes off to war. I could go on, but I think you get the point. I am sold on TOW and its benefits.

The scandal at Walter Reed had originally spurred me to act, planting the seed that ancient Greek war plays might somehow help service members and their families today. Three years later things had come full circle. The deputy commander of the First Infantry Division, awakened to action by Sophocles's plays, had returned to the source of my inspiration, Walter Reed, to demand more resources to address the mental health needs of soldiers, spouses, and families in his community. The plays had inspired a military leader to change his attitude toward the invisible wounds of war and, most important, to take action. When I was imagining the ten generals sitting in their thrones near the front of the Theater of Dionysus watching the premiere of Sophocles's *Ajax* unfold, I had always envisioned a similar reaction.

That night, after the performance of *Ajax* for spouses and families at the Fort Riley community center, I tried to unwind at the Holiday Inn. But many of the stories told by spouses stayed with me, echoing in my ears, invading my thoughts and my dreams. Over the past few months, I had grown accustomed to hearing dark, disturbing accounts of the aftermath of war. Although I had not become desensitized to these stories, they rarely caught me off guard anymore. But something about the sheer number of spouses that evening who had identified with Tecmessa's cries of despair—"Wretched, I am wretched!"—when she discovers the body of her dead husband, shook me to my core. "What am I to do now?" asks Tecmessa, standing over her husband's corpse. "Oh Ajax, this was no way to die, not for you. Even your enemies will weep when they see you."

PROMETHEUS IN SOLITARY

I

In the months following the first performance of Theater of War, I began thinking of other audiences that might be helped by ancient Greek tragedies. If Sophocles could be of service to those who served our country, then perhaps he and his contemporaries, Aeschylus and Euripides, could be put to work for other communities. As I began looking at the tragedies through the lens of prospective audiences, certain plays seemed as if they might have something important to say to people working in professions that brought them into close, daily contact with suffering and death, but who had no outlet for acknowledging the moral and emotional stress of their jobs. As the number of projects expanded, the ancient plays would lead me and my theater company, Outside the Wire, to audiences in prisons, churches, hospices, and homeless shelters, and these audiences would, in their responses, illuminate the real world relevance of the plays.

Aeschylus's *Prometheus Bound* tells the story of a god who was placed in solitary confinement, nailed to a cliff at the farthest reaches of the earth, for giving fire to man. In the spring of 2009, I set to work on translating *Prometheus Bound* with the goal of one day presenting it in correctional facilities. The more I read about mass incarceration, the more passionate I became about developing a project that would create the conditions for crucial dialogue within prisons. And the more time I spent with Aeschylus's ancient text, the stronger my conviction grew that it would resonate with people who worked in corrections.

Prometheus Bound, after all, is not a courtroom drama. It is an exploration of extreme incarceration, from the perspective not just of the prisoner but of the characters around him. Over the course of the play, Prometheus is visited by a series of characters for whom it is not difficult to find contemporary parallels: corrections officers (Kratos, Bia, and Hephaestus), social workers (Oceanus), aggrieved relatives (the Oceanids), and an assistant warden (Hermes), all of whom come to try to convince him to lower his head before the all-powerful warden in the sky, Zeus.

When I started working on the project we came to call "Prometheus in Prison," I had never set foot inside a prison, and I knew no one in the field of corrections. To test my theory about the play, I would need an audience. To find one, I would need to convince someone in charge of a prison or a prison system that performing the play for staff would be a worthwhile use of time and funds. In early June 2009, I landed my first audition for the project with the Missouri Department of Corrections.

"I've read the play, and I've gotta ask you, what do you hope to accomplish by performing it here?" Big John, a prison detective for the state of Missouri, was holding up the paperback Penguin Classics edition of Aeschylus's *Prometheus Bound* as if it were a piece of damning evidence.

It was a sweltering late-spring morning in Jefferson City. Beads of sweat were pooling on my brow, but I hesitated to wipe them away, for fear of raising further suspicion from this already skeptical crowd. On one side of a large rectangular conference table sat the entire executive staff of the Missouri Department of Corrections, glaring distrustfully in my direction. On the other sat George Lombardi, their boss. He was the one man in American corrections, I had been assured by Robin Mayer, my contact inside Rikers Island, the largest jail in New York City, who was "crazy" enough to entertain the idea of presenting Prometheus in Prison to his line staff. That would include corrections officers, social workers, food service employees, and custodians who worked long hours in the Missouri prisons. Few programs, if any, were geared toward their psychological well-being, and, according to Robin, George would likely see the value in any program designed for them.

Big John leaned forward in his dark suit, waving the translation in the air as he spoke, then paused to leaf suspiciously through the introduction. He looked over at me with his shifting, dark eyes. It seemed as if all the lights in the room had suddenly gone out, and he was shining a huge floodlight in my face, demanding that I defend Aeschylus's ancient play.

I hadn't expected such a hostile response, but it should not have come as a surprise. After all, many scholars consider *Prometheus Bound* to be one of the strongest condemnations of authoritarian rule, unjust imprisonment, and cruel and unusual punishment in all of Western literature. Prometheus, as Big John quickly pointed out, "gave fire to man," and from fire came everything we associate with being human. According to the myth, human consciousness itself could be traced back to Prometheus's crime, prior to which, according to one of Prometheus's more memorable speeches, humans stumbled through the dark, "unable to apprehend the true nature of anything they see."

Big John had a point. How could anyone who saw the play not feel moral outrage and antipathy toward Prometheus's captors? Also, as many in the room were quick to acknowledge, the media always, without fail, portray corrections officers as monsters, further isolating an already misunderstood profession.

Listening to Big John's argument, I began to question my own motives, as if about to confess to a crime I had yet to commit. I have always kept personal politics out of my work and tried to approach all audiences without judgment. But when it came to our overpopulated prison system, it was hard to remain unbiased. In 2011, according to the U.S. Department of Justice, there were "6.98 million offenders under the supervision of the adult correctional system," roughly one in every thirty-four adults. All told, that's 2.9 percent of the adult population. Of those, nearly 2.2 million men and women live behind bars in state and federal prisons.

And of those, roughly 25,000 are currently serving time in solitary confinement in supermax prisons, while somewhere between 50,000 and 80,000 more are living in "segregation units" and "restricted housing," which typically means solitary confinement. Though many corrections professionals in America maintain that isolation is a useful, humane tool, given the limited resources at their disposal, many psychologists and human rights activists consider the long-term practice of isolation tantamount to torture; many other first-world countries have all but abolished its prolonged use. It's difficult to talk about American corrections, and in particular solitary confinement, without taking a position or wading deep into political waters.

Also, my choice of play gave Big John every right to question my intentions. For centuries, Prometheus has been seen as the most iconic martyr of all time, a proto-Christian figure who suffered on behalf of humanity. Prometheus's punishment was a hideous form of torture. According to the legend, every morning the sun burned his skin to a crisp, and when night came, he was covered in frostbite. One myth even had it that a fierce eagle came each day to gorge itself on his liver, which regenerated overnight and was eaten again the next day. Prometheus was stripped of his dignity for helping humanity. Was there any way of interpreting or framing Aeschylus's play that wouldn't somehow feel like an indictment of the corrections system today?

Big John and the rest of the staff patiently waited for me to explain my purpose.

Prometheus Bound, I conceded, is a play about a god who is imprisoned for stealing fire from the gods and giving it to humans. But Prometheus admits that he willfully committed the crime as an act of political defiance. He violated the law and gave fire to humans in order to undermine the power of the new ruler—Zeus—during a period of political upheaval. But only days before, Prometheus had helped install Zeus, using his power to lock away his own family, the Titans, in the dark depths of Tartarus for all time. Prometheus was a double agent. His motives were conflicted, at best, when he helped humanity. And so the story of his crime and punishment, at least in Aeschylus's version, isn't aimed at eliciting our—i.e., human—sympathy. *Prometheus Bound* is a timeless story about power, surveillance, hierarchy, control, and—most important—martyrdom.

Looking up from the table, I could see that I had lost most of the executive staff's attention. Blank stares and quizzical looks permeated the conference room. So I redoubled my efforts.

Prometheus Bound is not a play about the ancient judicial process, I told them. It's about what happens to Prometheus once he's been locked away. Also, it's about gods, not humans. Think of the gods as corrections officers, I suggested. The world is a prison where humans are the inmates and gods hold all the power. Prometheus is like a corrections officer who plays favorites, or grants favors to the inmates, or lets down his guard, and gets into trouble for it, angering his peers. He broke the law and was sentenced severely for it, forced to live in isolation in a remote region of the Caucasus Mountains somewhere in Scythia for eternity. But the play doesn't concern itself with whether Zeus's law was just. Instead, it focuses on what happens to Prometheus, and how his behavior brings about even worse punishments once he enters the Olympian criminal justice system. Anyone working in corrections, I said, who has dealt with recalcitrant, angry, self-righteous, self-destructive prisoners like Prometheus will be able to relate to the power struggle in the play and some of the timeless issues it raises.

Big John stood down, but he didn't rest his case. He was far from convinced. If anything, the wordiness of my defense had set off alarms. Of course, his job was to root out the truth. I later learned that one of the executive staff members, a trusted colleague of George Lombardi, the director, had remarked to his colleagues after the meeting, "You know this sounds like Pandora's box. Do we really want to open Pandora's box?" Fortunately, none of the executives would be the final arbiter. The decision rested solidly in director George Lombardi's hands, and something told me that he had already made it.

George broke the silence. "I'm thinking we'll make this an optional event and host it off-site at the National Guard headquarters. Also, I'd like to offer continuing education credit to those who attend."

Heads nodded, if not in agreement, then in acceptance.

The previous night George Lombardi had personally driven his state vehicle to the St. Louis airport to pick me up. I could easily have spotted him in a lineup as a former warden: something about his size and how he carried himself, the combination of his viselike grip of a handshake and welcoming midwestern smile. He was a gentle giant who had mellowed with age, as his hair went gray and his ears grew hard of hearing. Governor Jay Nixon—a lone liberal in a sea of red—had pulled George out of retirement to run his prisons.

When I asked, on the two-hour ride to "Jeff City," if any good restaurants were still open, George looked at me incredulously and said, "Bryan, good, God-fearing people live in Jeff City, and they're all in bed. We roll up the sidewalks at eight p.m."

As we snaked down the dark highway, I learned that he had begun his career, straight out of school, as a prison psychologist, and that he had always been motivated by what he called the "rehabilitation of offenders."

"I'm interested in closing prisons," he said.

The Missouri system incarcerates roughly 30,000 prisoners, and employs 10,000 corrections workers to manage them. The average direct cost, per prisoner, is around $20,000 per year, and the average cost to build one prison is $120 million. Imagine, George suggested, if that money were spent instead on drug treatment, job training, or education.

Robin, a mental health counselor at Rikers Island and George's cousin, had been right. There was likely no individual in American corrections more open-minded than he.

While Missouri's prisoners were behind bars, George continued, they got good health care, both physical and psychological. But he chafed at the fact that after many state hospitals were shuttered in the 1970s, corrections had become the de facto mental-health-care system, not just in Missouri but throughout the country. "Most offenders get better care than the average Missouri citizen," he continued with unapologetic pride, going on to describe the cancer treatment and hospice programs that had been implemented during his tenure.

We pulled into a truck stop, and over omelets and home fries at a smoke-filled greasy spoon there, he laid out his vision for corrections in Missouri. "The system is divided into two groups—those who believe their job is to punish, and those who believe they're there to rehabilitate."

His approach was not revolutionary—he believed in slow, incremental change. Though he was ideologically opposed to the death penalty, he had presided over many executions. As a public servant, he saw it as his role to uphold the law, however morally repugnant he might find aspects of it. Yet using his position, he intended to change the system from within—not overnight, but over time. His objective was to return prisoners to their communities with the skills, support systems, and emotional stability to remain there. So he spent a good deal of his energy on reducing recidivism, which meant evangelizing for early childhood education as well as mental health and drug treatment programs.

George warned me that not all his staff members were as open-minded as he, especially at the executive level. Some thought that he had finally lost his mind when he invited me to fly from New York City to talk about performing a play by Aeschylus for corrections officers. But others saw the project as a natural extension of the programs he already supported as director—restorative justice initiatives, victims' classes in which violent criminals met with those they had harmed, vocational training, art studios, Web design workshops, agriculture programs, and even "Puppies for Parole," a rescue program for stray dogs in which prisoners participate in the dogs' rehabilitation, to name only a few. He had established himself as an outlier in the field of corrections, a leader in the struggle to reshape the criminal justice system rather than perpetuate the nineteenth-century penitentiary model.

The next morning, sitting across from Big John while he grilled me about *Prometheus,* I started to sense why my proposal seemed so threatening to the prison staff. From what I had observed so far, nearly everyone working in the criminal justice system seemed acutely aware of his or her prescribed role—and that they were all playing roles. Many of the corrections officers came from the same socioeconomic background as the prisoners, from similar neighborhoods, schools, and families. And many seemed to understand that a very thin barrier separated them from the population they kept locked up. However, there was no sanctioned occasion or place where this could be acknowledged.

It was not the job of corrections professionals, I mused, to question the law—their job was to enforce it. Also, in high-security settings, appearing to show softness or perceived weakness in front of prisoners could likely result in violent or even fatal consequences. I could see they all had feelings about injustices and inequities they witnessed and sometimes perpetrated, or didn't stop from being perpetrated, every day. For the most part, I suspected, they had to keep those thoughts to themselves, for fear of retribution from within their own ranks. Some most likely became bitter and, out of necessity, had purposefully drawn away or detached from their own emotions.

A corrections officer confirmed my suppositions when I spoke with him later. The principal reason the staff was so resistant to the idea of Prometheus in Prison, he explained, was that "a lot of people are afraid of retribution. If they spoke up in a meeting about what happened to them, or with their supervisors, they'd be afraid they would get retaliated against."

Perhaps what was most threatening about my presence, that morning in Missouri, wasn't the play itself but the permission the play would give to people working in this deeply challenging profession to speak truthfully about the distress they felt every day simply doing their jobs. Big John and his colleagues could tell I wasn't there to point fingers or spit invective from the stage, or to subversively undermine George Lombardi's authority. They saw that I had come with good intentions. But they were worried that creating a forum for corrections staff to vent what had been pent up inside them would have unintended consequences. What would happen when we took the lid off the pressure cooker? Would the line staff explode with anger and complaints? Or could something constructive and even healing come from open dialogue?

My work with the military suggested that corrections staff would likely find relief in hearing others articulate their private inner conflicts. And from what I had read and heard about corrections, prison was clearly dehumanizing for everyone inside, both guards and guarded. But in the end, it would be impossible for me to know how corrections staff would react to the play until the first performance.

I I

Later that same morning George drove me over to the Central Missouri Corrections Center, a maximum-security facility ten miles south of downtown Jefferson City. A man named Dave, with a red handlebar mustache, a firm handshake, and a cool, steady gaze, greeted us in the lobby. He was the warden, and he seemed right out of central casting—not for a prison film but for a classic Western. He had the distant, weathered look of a sheriff who never flinched when the bullets flew.

We checked our cell phones at the front desk and were waved through a series of metal gates and tight antechambers. Finally, a thick steel door slammed ominously behind us, and all of a sudden we were "inside the wire," as it is called in corrections. Dave led us past a towering electric fence, which George casually remarked had been installed after an attempted prison break; the fence was expensive, but it was 100 percent effective and had reduced the number of staff members needed to guard the facility's perimeter. Whenever an unlucky bird chanced to land on the new electric fence, he said, corrections officers would hear a loud pop and see a dark plume of smoke hovering over the coils. Anything living would be vaporized. Nothing remained but charred feathers and mangled claws.

We walked through an open courtyard, past the fogged-up windows of a cafeteria packed with inmates shoveling colorless, tasteless food products into their mouths. We passed rows of tiny classrooms in which seasoned convicts, poised before whiteboards like college professors, led seminars aimed at "cultivating compassion" for victims of violent crimes. Some of these classes, George remarked, resulted in face-to-face meetings between inmates and their victims.

In cases of murder, the meetings could involve members of the victim's family and would be organized largely for their benefit. The murderer would apologize, at length, take responsibility for the crime, and explain how, during his long years of incarceration, he had begun to comprehend the pain he had inflicted, the sorrow and immeasurable loss that had resulted from his actions. The goal was not to achieve forgiveness but to help bring closure to the victims' families. According to George, the sessions could be very emotional for all parties, exemplifying the power of restorative justice to heal both the offender and the victim.

As I listened to him, I tried my best to keep an open mind. Even if compassion classes seemed idealistic, and slightly Orwellian, that approach was far preferable to straight incarceration.

Dave swiped a key and a door swung open, revealing a long, narrow corridor. Men in drab uniforms filed past us in no apparent hurry. They did not, as I had imagined, bear the telltale look of the condemned, like the men described in Kafka's *The Trial*. We could have been walking through the hallway of a Title I school, a public hospital, or an army barracks. The prison seemed orderly, at least on the surface, though George had warned me in his understated manner that "incidents do happen." In the presence of these docile, seemingly innocuous men, I momentarily forgot about the types of crimes that had led to their incarceration. They seemed ordinary and unthreatening.

I asked George if inmates were categorized and grouped by the nature of their crimes—murderers with murderers, rapists with rapists. He unequivocally replied that his aim was to ensure that all offenders were treated equally, by staff and by one another. And so their crimes were not made known, even to corrections officers. (This happens to be, as I later learned, a general rule in American prisons.) Also, neither class nor race affected how the staff treated inmates, at least in principle. All religions were welcome. Prisoners served time on equal footing regardless of their crimes. Inmates were defined not by what they had done on the outside but by how they behaved inside the electric fence. As if to illustrate this point, George turned to me and asked, "Are you ready to meet Prometheus?"

Minutes later we entered the "administrative segregation" unit, a euphemism for solitary confinement. From a distance, I heard men shouting, a cacophony of voices calling out for human contact reverberating through the central corridor. The building, which had clearly been built for surveillance, featured a command center with tinted black windows and banks of blinking black-and-white closed-circuit screens, monitored 24/7 by a rotating staff of corrections officers. A handful of long, narrow hallways radiated out from the all-seeing nerve center, like the arms of a starfish.

As we approached, the shouting and howling grew louder. Some of the prisoners seemed to be talking to the voices in their heads, others communicated with one another, while still others berated the corrections officers with questions and complaints. Though the voices differed in tone and pitch, they had a unity of purpose: all were speaking with the same voice of recalcitrance and dissent—the voice of Prometheus. I recognized it from Aeschylus's play. Was this what George had meant?

When Prometheus's relatives, the Oceanids, first come to visit him on the cliff, he questions their intentions with a mixture of sarcasm, derision, and suspicion:

PROMETHEUS
Why have you come?
To see me suffering?

Where did
you find
the courage
to leave
behind your
home, your
caves carved
from sandstone
by cold streams
to visit this land-
locked strip mine?

Perhaps you
have come
to witness
the crimes
that have been
perpetrated
against me?

Perhaps you have
come to share
in the misery
by quietly
observing
my pain?
Then get a good look.

That morning inside the administrative segregation unit, I felt that anyone who saw me there would have harbored similar suspicions. The unit hummed with a dark, manic energy, an unnameable tension, like a strange vibration—an electromagnetic field tightening in my chest.

Dave conferred quietly with a guard, who then opened a door to a hallway that snaked out from the nerve center. We passed several small cells, stopping briefly to peer inside, as if searching for chameleons in a terrarium hiding against rocks in plain sight. It was hard to make out much through the slim windows, but in each cell lived a man who had been quarantined for an indefinite period of time. Most of them would spend twenty-three hours a day in confinement, with a single hour to shower or exercise—still alone—in metal cages.

I heard Prometheus before I saw him. The words were garbled and unclear, but he said something about being "allergic to beans," and I was startled to discover just how physically close we were to the man who spoke these words. He wasn't languishing in one of the isolation chambers, cut off from humanity. He was inches away, within arm's reach.

The man moved forward, out of the shadows and into the light. The whites of his eyes flashed, illuminating bristly black hair and an unkempt beard. He was shivering and naked, standing in a shower—or more accurately, a cage with a spigot—dripping wet, without a towel. Neither of my guides attempted to interpret what I was looking at; nor did they apologize or try to justify in any way what happened next. They just let it happen.

With a sudden glint of recognition in his eyes, the prisoner saw who was standing before him and realized that he had—against all odds—finally been granted a personal audience with those in power. Without hesitation, he began to argue his case with a steady stream of words, shouting at the top of his lungs, through the bars, about the injustice of his suffering. He said he'd been deprived of food for seventeen days. All that time, the guards had only brought him beans. They knew he was allergic to beans and were trying to murder him, starve him to death and make it look as if he had refused to eat. He hadn't been allowed to shave or bathe, either. He had rights, he insisted. What about his rights?

During the inmate's monologue, at once both a powerful prosecution and an impassioned defense, Dave remained stoically unfazed. Then the outburst abated, and the prisoner paused, briefly, to catch his breath.

As I listened to his well-wrought arguments, I

couldn't help but hear the righteously indignant voice
of Prometheus, defending his actions and condemning
his captors:

PROMETHEUS
I saved men
from total
annihilation,
from almost
certain Death
and now I am
to endure
these terrible
tortures, painful
to feel, almost
worse to observe.

I treated men
with compassion,
but was not thought
worthy enough
to receive it in return.

Instead, I will
be displayed for
all to see,
so ruthlessly
abused that
even Zeus
averts his eyes.

> My punishment
> is a disgrace
> to the one who
> punishes me.

Like the prisoner in question, Prometheus makes a compelling argument about the injustice of his incarceration, one that is hard to refute. As Dave watched the prisoner, I wondered what he would say to the man's many complaints. Dave stepped forward, never breaking contact with the prisoner's fiery eyes, and calmly replied, "Let me ask you this. Why did you get to take a shower today?" He hadn't been deprived of food. As it turned out, the man inside the cage had just ended a hunger strike. As a reward, he had been offered a shower.

Everything that takes place within an American prison is based on a system of rewards and punishments or, in psychological terms, positive and negative reinforcement. In many prisons, a prisoner who does not violate the rules is granted access to a wide array of privileges, living among other prisoners in a highly regimented community but watched at every turn. However, every time a prisoner breaks the rules, privileges are taken away, including social contact with other prisoners. Therefore, as Dave later explained, the staff is interested in whether prisoners obey the rules, not in what they say about them. The corrections staff don't care about rhetoric, no matter how compelling, or about what prisoners had done to get locked up in the first place. Inside the prison, behavior matters most.

In many cases, George said, prisoners are placed in administrative segregation because they are considered candidates for acts of violence; they are segregated to protect the general prison population. Other prisoners are there to be protected from others who wanted to perpetrate acts of violence upon them. Lamentably, many prisoners in segregation struggle with underlying mental health issues, which are exacerbated by isolation. They are effectively being punished for being sick, which makes them more ill.

The unnamed arguing prisoner was a convicted criminal who had been incarcerated for a serious, possibly violent, crime, but his words touched my heart and awakened my moral outrage at what I perceived to be the indignity of his condition. I had been opposed to solitary confinement prior to seeing it with my own eyes. After hearing the prisoner's voice, I was deeply shaken and searched within myself for the courage to speak out on his behalf. His short, emotionally charged monologue had completely swayed me to his side. But his words were meaningless to the warden. All that mattered was that he had eaten the beans.

The ancient Athenians were more inclined to impose penalties upon criminals than to incarcerate them. Technically, they did have jails, or holding cells, where the accused awaited trial and sentencing, such as the famous cell where Socrates was kept during the legal proceedings that led to his death, immortalized in Plato's dialogues. And those poor souls who were unable to pay their fines could be penalized with imprisonment. Some convicts were publicly humiliated; others were stripped of their political rights and property. But for the most part, the convicted were either exiled or executed. Athenian society had no need for the mass, long-term warehousing of men.

Some scholars believe that the courts and jails may have been emptied during the City Dionysia, the annual spring theater festival. The prisoners were released on bail—furloughed, so to speak—in order to attend the performances. Like everyone else, they would have been charged admission, which was minimal. However, if they did not have enough money to pay, they would be admitted for free. Given all this, it seems possible, even plausible, that those awaiting sentence, as well as their adjudicators, were present in the audience for the premiere of Aeschylus's *Prometheus* trilogy,* which included *Prometheus Bound*, about his captivity; *Prometheus Unbound*, about his release; and *Prometheus the Fire Bringer*, which was likely about his reintegration and reconciliation with the gods. Of these three plays, only *Prometheus Bound* has survived.

---

* There is little agreement among scholars regarding the dating of *Prometheus Bound*. Some even speculate that the play was not written by Aeschylus at all. For the purposes of clarity and continuity in this book, I will refer to it as Aeschylus's work, without staking a claim in the larger argument.

Today's large-scale imprisonment of criminals has no classical analogue, but solitary confinement has one in the practice of exile, an isolating punishment based on the deprivation of contact with other humans and, often, one's native language. Greek laws about exile were harsh and unforgiving. The exiled were expelled from their cities, stripped of their property and rights, and banned from athletic games and religious ceremonies; after death their remains could not be buried in their cities of origin. During their sentences they would become *metics,* or wandering migrants, with no claim to citizenship in their homeland. They would be cast out of society, removed from everyone and everything that was familiar.

Ancient Athens reserved exile primarily for the worst of crimes, such as homicide, for it was seen as a punishment worse than execution. According to fifth-century-BC Athenian law, the only way someone who committed involuntary manslaughter could be permitted to return from exile was to make peace with the relatives of his victim.

I should note that banishment in Athens was meted out to more than just criminals. People who were deemed for political reasons to be a threat to the state or to the fabric of democracy were also cast out of the city, usually for ten years, through a process called ostracism. Athenian citizens would meet annually to vote with pieces of broken pottery, or *ostraca,* on which they would scratch the names of individuals thought to be dangerous to the polis. The person with the most votes was ostracized. Ostracism was an extrajudicial, and many times preemptive, process that had nothing to do with criminal justice, but the result was much the same as exile.

Today prisoners serving long terms in isolation are, in effect, exiled from humanity. They are stripped of their rights, removed from society, and often denied contact with family and friends. The longer inmates are segregated and deprived of being spoken to or touched, the harder it is for them to reintegrate or socialize once they are released back into the general prison population or into society. Solitary confinement robs prisoners of their ability to connect with others. The longer they live in solitary confinement, the harder it is for them to return home.

The French philosopher Michel Foucault, in his landmark book *Discipline and Punish: The Birth of the Prison,* wrote, "Solitude is the primary condition of total submission." Standing in the administrative segregation unit in the Jefferson City Correctional Center, located at 8200 No More Victims Road, I could see that submission was indeed the intended goal, though it seemed equally clear that this type of long-term isolation would have far-reaching unintended consequences for the men inside.

Psychologists who study the behavior of inmates, prisoners of war, and hostages have long concluded that keeping people locked up in isolation is profoundly damaging. As the physician and writer Atul Gawande pointed out in a 2009 *New Yorker* article, "One of the paradoxes of solitary confinement is that, as starved as people become for companionship, the experience typically leaves them unfit for social interaction." The psychologist Craig Haney, he notes, studied the impact of isolation upon one hundred randomly selected inmates at a supermax facility in California. After months or years of solitary confinement, a large number of prisoners began "to lose the ability to initiate behavior of any kind—to organize their lives around activity and purpose." Moreover, "chronic apathy, lethargy, depression, and despair often result" from long-term isolation. "In extreme cases, prisoners may literally stop behaving, becoming essentially catatonic." Perhaps this is what Foucault meant by "total submission." If isolation strips prisoners of their ability to socialize, or in some cases to do anything at all, how can it be in the best interests of our country when at least 95 percent of all prisoners will ultimately be released and return to society?

Prometheus gave fire to humans and was punished with solitary confinement. In one way, his incarceration epitomizes the extreme of imposed isolation or exile, for he was a god, and gods are immortal: a life sentence naturally carries more weight for those who will never die. Condemned to live forever, nailed to the side of a cliff at the end of the earth, Prometheus elicits sympathy from anyone who hears his story. But at its core, I believe *Prometheus Bound* is about discipline and power within a complex hierarchy, not a one-sided condemnation of authoritarian rule. And it was for this reason that I imagined it would resonate with people who worked in corrections today.

Prometheus argues that his crime was one of conscience: he stole fire from the gods and gave it to humans. At the precise moment when Zeus wished to exterminate humanity, Prometheus offered up his freedom to save it. But a quick examination of the backstory reveals Prometheus to be a duplicitous character, a trickster with no moral center, who acts not in accordance with his conscience but to serve his own interests and desires.

Each character in the play who visits Prometheus imparts advice about how he can reduce the severity of his sentence, but their advice falls on increasingly deaf ears. The longer his incarceration lasts, the more self-isolating and self-destructive Prometheus becomes. The more isolated he feels, the more compelled he is to kick, goad, threaten, taunt, and provoke his jailers until he is made to suffer punishments beyond his fertile and prophetic imagination. Like a prisoner who refuses to eat in order to exercise control over a situation in which he finds himself otherwise powerless, Prometheus rails against Zeus and his minions with the hope of exposing the corruption of those who have imprisoned him.

In the last scene of the play, he digs in his heels and redoubles his indignation and rage, hoping to trigger a reaction in his captors, daring them to punish him even more.

PROMETHEUS
So let the lightning
lash me from above;
let mighty thunder
rattle the heavens
and whip up the gales;
let a swirling storm
uproot the earth and
send giant waves
cresting skyward
into the orbits of
the stars and spheres;
let him pick up my
broken body and
cast it into the dark-
ness of Tartarus.

I will stand in the eye
of the storm, staring
down Necessity,
but my spirit shall
never be broken.

Prometheus spends the play's final moments cursing
Zeus and mocking him with prophecies of his eventual
downfall, which he doggedly refuses to explain, even
under the threat of torture. After his death, he is buried,
like his brothers the Titans, under a mountain of rock,
while calling out to his mother—Earth—and the "all-
seeing sun" to "witness the injustice of [his] suffering."

Prometheus Bound raises profound questions about what happens inside prisons—or for that matter, inside any institution that maintains order through surveillance and punishment. Why does a prisoner seem bent on self-destruction? Who wins when he is, so to speak, buried under rocks? And how do we get angry, self-righteous, rebellious prisoners out from under the rocks and back into society? I hoped the line staff of the Missouri Department of Corrections would feel compelled to answer such questions after watching scenes from Aeschylus's play. But later that summer, when we finally performed it in Jefferson City, the audience—ranging from food service workers to wardens—steered the conversation in unexpected directions, defying all my expectations.

"Who is Prometheus? Have you seen him? Worked with him?" I asked the crowd of roughly two hundred corrections staff members.

"I see him every day," offered a dispirited social worker, who went on to enumerate the countless challenges of attempting to reach angry, defiant prisoners, and often failing to move the needle.

"Okay. Who is Zeus?"

"Zeus is the eighty-five percent rule," someone blurted out, referring to the harsh, across-the-board Missouri mandate that inmates convicted of dangerous felonies serve 85 percent of any sentence before being considered for parole.

"Zeus is mandatory minimum drug-sentencing laws," chimed someone else.

"Zeus is when fathers default on alimony payments and are kept in prison because of it."

"Zeus," said an angry-looking corrections officer in the front, pointing his finger straight at my chest, "is that if both of us were charged with a DUI, you would get off lightly and I would get time."

Zeus, it seemed, was not a brutal dictator or some warden in the sky. To the corrections staff, he, and his seemingly unjust treatment of Prometheus, was a metaphor for all the inequalities and injustices within the criminal justice system. Big John, the prison detective who now sat off to the left, eyeing me from the front row, had been right. The audience had reflexively sympathized with Prometheus. Some even identified with him.

"I'm Prometheus," offered a corrections officer. "I can be disciplined for the choices I make each day. If I make the wrong choice, I could end up behind bars."

"I'm Prometheus," echoed another corrections officer in the back. "The only difference is that I serve time eight hours a day."

At the end of the discussion, which continued for over an hour, George Lombardi offered closing remarks. He spoke passionately and eloquently about how much he believed in the profession of corrections and in the ability of the people gathered in the auditorium to make a difference in the lives of prisoners, their families, and their communities.

Then, after warm applause, he asked the actors and

me to remain on stage to be recognized. He placed a square stone in each actor's hand. "To show our appreciation," he said, "these are from the wall of the old state penitentiary." They had been engraved with the actors' names. He then reached behind the podium and pulled out a small statue, extending it to me. "And this is a statue of Prometheus that was carved by one of our offenders."

The sculpture was stunning—it featured a tortured, contorted Prometheus nailed to the side of a cliff, pulling at his chains. It had clearly taken months to complete. (The man who made it, an elderly prisoner, I was later told, died not long after the performance. Sadly, I never got the chance to meet him or to thank him.) As we were walking out of the venue, Big John, who had been sitting silently in the front row, walked over and shook my hand with a crushing grip. "You were right," he said with thinly veiled incredulity, as if he still couldn't believe it.

That December, George Lombardi invited us to return, this time to perform in a women's correctional facility in Vandalia, Missouri. We cast the fierce New York actress Elizabeth Marvel in the lead role and called it Promethea in Prison. Elizabeth gave a chilling performance, tearing into the text, shedding rivers of tears, and wailing at the top of her lungs for someone to witness her suffering.

When the performance was over, toward the end of the audience discussion, a heavyset female guard shouted out, "I want to know how Elizabeth knew what it sounds like when women are dragged to the hole." Elizabeth slid down in her chair, embarrassed to be asked such a direct question, and quietly replied that it had been her first time inside a prison.

"Why do you ask?" I interjected in an attempt to save Elizabeth from further questioning.

"Men always go silently," the woman responded, wringing her meaty hands, "but women always go kicking and screaming."

Heads nodded in agreement, and a hush fell over the room, as if some secret, universal truth about human nature had been let out of the bag.

III

One of the corrections officers at the Jefferson City premiere who seemed most affected by the performance was an imposingly large captain in his late fifties. George Adkinson wore thick Coke-bottle glasses that magnified his penetrating stare. From the minute we met, after the executive session that spring, Captain Adkinson had opened up to me, in a pure, unrehearsed way. It was as if he had been waiting his entire life for someone to ask him about his experiences working in prisons, and I just happened to be the first.

Adkinson had not always known he would be a corrections officer, or that he would spend much of his adult life behind bars. The events that led to his landing a job in the old Missouri State Penitentiary seem to him, in retrospect, to have unfolded by chance. He could just

as easily have ended up working on a farm, or for the
military at nearby Fort Leonard Wood, or managing the
gas station in the little rural town of Richland, where
he was hired out of high school, thanks to his father-
in-law. But after graduating in 1970 and marrying his
sweetheart, Adkinson found himself struggling to make
ends meet while his wife attended nursing school. He
simply couldn't make enough to pay the bills.

One day when he was twenty-two, a good friend who
worked as a highway patrolman offered to put him forward for a job. But Adkinson wore glasses, and when
he revealed to his interviewer that he couldn't meet the
patrol's requirement of seeing 20/30 without them, he
had to give up any aspiration of becoming a highway
patrolman. For the next two years, he and his wife
remained in Richland until a good friend persuaded
him to drive up to the penitentiary in Jefferson City and
put in an application.

At the interview, a young man named Mel Gardner who managed personnel at the prison looked over
Adkinson's file. "George, have you ever been convicted
of a felony?" he asked.

"No, sir, I have not."

"How come?" Gardner asked.

"Probably because I've never been caught," Adkinson deadpanned.

As it turned out, Gardner had also grown up in rural
Missouri and understood that only the grace of God
separated those who worked in the penitentiary from
those who served time there. He must have appreci-

ated the candor of Adkinson's response, because a few weeks later, Adkinson got a call instructing him when and where to report for his first day.

The old Missouri State Penitentiary, which was erected in 1868, was replete with gothic stonework, gas chambers, and crumbling cells, resembling a medieval dungeon more than a modern correctional facility. On Adkinson's first day on the job, the metal gates slammed behind him with a thunderous sound, as he was locked inside the inner walls of the prison. *Oh my gosh,* he thought, *what have I gotten myself into? Here I am, a country boy from a small town of eleven hundred people, and I'm up in this penitentiary that's got twenty-five hundred felons in it. What have I done?*

Over the following two weeks, as he acclimated to his new work environment, he began to observe that "most" of the inmates there "were just trying to do their time and go home." They kept their heads down and stayed out of trouble: "Even back then, when corrections was considered a place just to warehouse the worst of society, to get 'em out, they still had that one goal of getting back home." In spite of its intimidating, draconian-looking exterior, the Missouri State Penitentiary turned out to be a community where a majority of the inhabitants abided by the law and lived peacefully.

After a few months of working inside and walking "hand in hand, shoulder to shoulder" with the inmates, "ninety-nine percent of the time I didn't feel any more threatened walking among them than I did walking down a crowded street." The longer Adkinson worked there, the less difference he saw between the world within the towering stone walls and the world outside. "A lot of people have misconceptions of prison," he told me. "A prison's like a city with walls. . . . And it has the same problems that any big city does: it has murder, it has violence, robbery, rapes—on a day-to-day basis." The difference was that inside the prison, the corrections officers were the protectors of the population and the enforcers of the law.

In spite of the fact that the inmates kept their living quarters fairly clean, there was always a strong, penetrating, unpleasant smell inside the prison, "a combination of body odor, burnt food, and disinfectant." It remained with Adkinson, on his uniform and in his pores, for hours after he left work: "Many times when I'd come home my wife would make me take off my clothes in the garage because the smell just stuck to me. It was horrible. And people don't believe me when I tell 'em that the air smelled different inside the walls than it did outside. But it did."

The noxious smell wasn't the only thing Adkinson brought home from work. He was developing a tough-guy persona. "They always tell you to leave it at the door when you leave and pick it back up when you come back in, but I couldn't. After you're there for a while, it gets ingrained in you." Corrections officers, and law enforcement in general, have a high divorce rate, which he attributes to the attitude that they have to assume at work. Over time it doesn't come off as easily as the uniform. "Unfortunately," he said, "you bring that home, and that stays with you. I can't tell you the number of times my first wife told me to quit talking to her like a convict. Even after I was married to my second wife, even though I'd been retired, I still had that hateful, cynical attitude." After he retired in 2010, "it took me about a year to finally mellow out enough, to where every answer I would give my wife didn't have a hateful tone to it, like 'What are you asking me that for? Are you stupid?'—you know. Yeah, it sticks with you. You take it home with you. No matter how hard you try, you can't leave it at work."

Near the end of his career, after more than thirty-three years of working inside the correctional system, after all the accumulated stress that came with the job, Adkinson finally burned out and lost his drive. He said to himself one day, "I've grown old in this penitentiary. It's made me old before my time. It's cost me my health. It's cost me my wife. I'm done."

Regarding inmates, Adkinson reflected, "it's all in the way you treat 'em. If you show 'em respect, you're gonna get respect back from 'em. If you don't show 'em respect, you're not gonna get any respect back from 'em." In all his time working in prison, he was never assaulted, in large part due to his approach. Over his career, however, he witnessed his fair share of situations in which officers lost control of inmates. He likened these experiences to combat. "We're constantly puttin' ourselves in harm's way," he said. "We fight a different war than today's soldiers. Instead of with bullets and bombs, our enemy fights back with verbal abuse, with feces, with spit, with stabbings in the cells. But you know, we fight the same wars, just on different ground."

One incident remains indelibly seared in his memory, causing him to relive the helplessness and the horror. "It happened over at the old penitentiary," he said. "I was a lieutenant on the morning watch. I was getting ready to go home, and I was briefing the day shift captain on anything that happened that night. Right above the captain's office was housing unit five.

"Suddenly, we heard the sergeant call ten-five, which means 'I need help quick.' So all of us who were in the captain's office, we all ran out there. Two inmates were fighting at the bottom of the steps. One had a knife, and the other one didn't have anything but his fists. Long story short, the inmate that had the knife ended up killing the other one. And after the last stab, he motioned with his hands to say 'I'm done with him.'

"So we opened the gate that was separating us, and we pulled the dead inmate in. Well, as soon as he fell to the floor, it was just like a five-gallon bucket of blood gushed out of his chest. The inmate had ended up stabbing him forty-three times, and two of 'em struck through the heart. So not only me but several of us watched this man get stabbed to death.

"I didn't sleep for three days. And my wife, bless her heart, she tried to understand what I was going through, but she didn't know. She was a registered nurse; she sees death all the time. I don't see death that often. So yeah, that really bothered me. And even to this day, if I let my mind go, I can see that replay over and over and over again."

The first time Adkinson saw the actor Bill Camp embody the role of Prometheus, the intensity of the performance brought him right back to that moment when the gushing blood poured forth from the stabbed man, filling him with an inexplicable sense of panic and fear. Listening to Prometheus howl in pain and feeling helpless in the face of his agony reminded Adkinson of what it had been like to stand on the other side of the gate watching the stabbing.

After the incident, Adkinson had desperately wanted to talk to someone, anyone, about what happened, but there were no psychological services available for corrections officers at that time: "Nobody outside other than my wife wanted to hear about it." So he swept his memories under the rug and tried to get back to work. The discussion after the performance in Jefferson City was his first opportunity to tell the story in a large, open setting, to a receptive audience. Though the images would always be with him, by talking about what he saw, he finally managed to get something off his chest that had been weighing on him for years.

Adkinson knew the social stigma of working in prisons firsthand. He remembered a "well-known radio personality" saying on his local talk show, "If you wanna see the scum of the earth, just stand out in front of the

Missouri State Penitentiary shift change." That remark stuck with him over the years. And when he told people what he did for a living, he was often met with silent judgment. Nearly every portrayal of prison life, in television and movies, depicts corrections officers as "corrupt idiots."

Yet from his perspective nothing could have been further from the truth. His profession subjected him to isolation and unique pressures. "I've been in situations where I felt like I was Prometheus and everybody had abandoned me," he said. In fact, the idea of Prometheus as a corrections officer struck him as a more fitting analogy than Prometheus as an inmate. Prometheus, in his estimation, got into trouble for showing inappropriate compassion for humans. A corrections officer could easily end up in that position for doing the same. Like Prometheus, corrections staff lived under the constant threat of harsh legal punishment if they in any way bent the rules for inmates.

As Adkinson saw it, Prometheus was a corrections officer who had done what he thought was right for the inmates under his supervision, but in doing so he had violated the warden's rules and was punished for it. He became an inmate himself and was sentenced to administrative segregation.

Regarding the use of isolation as a way of dealing with troublesome or recalcitrant inmates, Adkinson expressed mixed feelings. "Unfortunately," he said, "corrections facilities have limited resources at their disposal to use, and isolation is a tool." He had seen it break inmates and initiate positive change in their behavior. After a period, "they'll actually realize that they're the problem and that that's why they're in there, and they'll adjust their attitude, and they'll be fine the rest of their time in the penitentiary." But other inmates, those who behaved like Prometheus, seemed agitated and emboldened by the experience of isolation. "Some of 'em," Adkinson said, "are never gonna change. They might straighten up enough to work their way out of administrative segregation, but just as soon as they're out in the population, a month or two or six months down the road, they're gonna do something to go right back in it."

And a good number of inmates "function better when isolated," he said, because separated from the general prison population, they get the individualized attention they crave. And those who screamed the loudest, who kicked and banged on their doors, who refused to give back their food trays after meals, or who went on hunger strike, were sometimes more isolated out in the general prison population than they were in administrative segregation. Their extreme behavior "was just their way of getting attention" that they weren't getting, either from fellow inmates or staff.

Looking back on his career, Adkinson often wonders if he made a difference in the lives of the inmates. Unfortunately, because of the nature of corrections, officers like him see mainly the repeat offenders: "That's one of the things that makes the job so frustrating— you constantly see so many familiar faces coming back through." But the abiding belief that he was making a positive difference in some of the inmates' lives was what kept him coming back, clocking into work, day after day, year after year. "Maybe all these guys needed was somebody to talk to, to listen to them. And maybe something I said to 'em made a difference and helped them stay out. We just never know. I can count on one hand the number of inmates that came up to me and said, 'Hey, captain, back in 1989 that thing you said or did made a world of difference.'"

One time, however, he did run into an ex-felon on the street in Jefferson City, who said, "Hey, cap, you remember me? You were my CO when I was in the old penitentiary. I lived in housing unit three-A, cell twenty-five. . . . You were nice to me. I just wanna thank you for that." Moments like that make Adkinson's time inside the penitentiary seem worth it. "Thirty years have gone by. You know, I've seen so many faces, it's hard to recognize the ones that maybe didn't give me any trouble. You always remember the ones that gave you trouble; but the ones that didn't, you hardly ever remember 'em 'cause they never made an impression on ya. So yeah, every now and then you get that little shot of 'Hey, you know, maybe all those years paid off for somebody.'"

IV

When I began directing readings of Aeschylus's *Prometheus Bound* in prisons, I never dreamed of performing in the detention camps of Guantánamo Bay, Cuba. I had failed to gain access to Rikers Island, where I originally intended to pilot the project, and it had been hard enough to persuade the Missouri Department of Corrections to host performances for prison staff. The idea of performing at one of the most controversial military bases in American history, and persuading the four-star general who commanded the Southern Hemisphere to make Aeschylus's play mandatory viewing for guards in the camps, was not even a distant fantasy.

But six months after the Jefferson City premiere of Prometheus in Prison, we presented a Theater of War performance of *Ajax* for a large crowd of enlisted Marines at Camp Pendleton in Southern California. There, an ambitious young navy psychologist, Lieutenant Jason Duff, came up and shook my hand, pressed his card firmly into my palm, and mentioned in passing that he would soon be stationed at Gitmo.

Almost a year later, Lieutenant Duff called me—he had somehow persuaded a rear admiral to bring Theater of War to Guantánamo Bay. Morale was running low at the base, which at the time housed more than 5,500 troops, including many who had fought in the wars in Iraq and Afghanistan, and the leadership there was hoping the project might get service members and their families to open up and share their stories.

So that spring my producing partner Phyllis Kaufman and I and a group of Broadway actors boarded a charter flight in Miami, took a circuitous, three-hour trip around Cuban airspace over glistening aquamarine waters, and landed on the southeastern tip of the mysterious island. We presented performances of Sophocles's *Ajax* and *Philoctetes* in two large outdoor amphitheaters, for service members and their families. Based on the success of that first tour, less than six months later we were invited back, this time to present readings of scenes from *Prometheus Bound* for the guards.

The most unsettling part about visiting Gitmo is how normal everything seems, especially on the naval side of the base. A little American village at the mouth of Guantánamo Bay has been in existence since 1903, when the United States first leased the land to establish its naval installation. (Apparently we still send a check every year to the Castros, who purportedly keep the uncashed checks in a top desk drawer.) The naval side of the base features a golf course, a coffee shop, a library, a PX, a Subway, a Church's Fried Chicken, a chapel, an Irish pub, a marina, an elementary school, a movie theater, a cafeteria, a community center, a tiki bar, and an officers' club. A large, stately admiral's mansion sits on a cliff at the edge of the installation, surrounded by crystal-clear waters and gorgeous white-sand beaches, populated by iguanas and banana rats. An unfriendly Communist country lies just outside the borders of the perimeter fence.

Gitmo is a Joint Task Force, which is to say that it houses service members from the army, navy, air force, marines, and coast guard. A high-security area on the other side of the base, called Camp Delta, houses detainees from foreign countries behind razor wire; the United States is holding them indefinitely—without due process—as "enemy combatants." At one point, early in Camp Delta's existence, it housed more than nine hundred detainees.

But fewer than 150 men live there now. They have been languishing there for years, because other countries have refused to receive them or the United States deems them too dangerous to be released or, for that matter, to be tried on American soil. As you enter Camp Delta, a banner overhead displays the motto "Honor Bound to Protect Freedom." But the continued existence of Camp Delta has, in the eyes of many throughout the world, denigrated the very values it claims to uphold. Within a few hours of visiting the camps, the words *honor, bound,* and *freedom* all began to take on new significance for me.

On day two of our first visit, we were taken on a tour of Camp Delta. Before entering the more relaxed detention facilities, called Camp 6, modeled after a medium-security prison, we were brought to the adjoining hospital, where detainees receive medical treatment by an on-site staff of doctors, mental health professionals, and nurses who are assigned to administer only to them. We were led down a long, sterile corridor into a treatment room, where our tour guide, one of the medical officers at the hospital with an unsettlingly sanguine demeanor and an eerily broad smile, held up a can of Ensure—a feeding supplement—on a steel tray. Alongside the can rested a small white feeding tube.

In the name of transparency, the medical staff wished

to address up front one of the most controversial ethical issues: namely, the force-feeding of detainees who
go on hunger strike. The American Medical Association and the American Civil Liberties Union, along with
many other human rights organizations, have publicly
condemned the practice. Our guide handed me the tube
and passed around the can of liquid nutrition. He then
spoke about the protocols that had been put in place for
determining when a detainee who had gone on hunger
strike was in danger of precipitating his own death and
therefore was in need of forced feedings.

One of the actors asked about the frequency of hunger strikes and suicide attempts, and we learned that for
a large portion of the remaining detainees, the threat
of both was constant; hence the hypervigilance of both
the medical and the detention staffs. The last detainee
who killed himself, the camp's commanding officer told
us, had done so by fashioning "a noose out of candy
wrappers." Following that suicide, if any detainee was
suspected of posing a threat to himself or to others, he
would be placed in isolation, and three guards would
be assigned to watch over him, in fifteen-minute incre-
ments, twenty-four hours a day. Every three minutes, we
learned, a camera was pointed at every detainee in the
camp. The facility had been designed for total surveillance. Three minutes, we were told, is how long it takes
for someone to die by strangulation.

After our brief visit in the hospital, we were led
through the dimly lit inner corridor of Camp 6, which
permitted us to peer through two-way mirrors without

being detected by the detainees. Knowing that politicians and dignitaries often walked the halls, the detainees had placed signs of protest against the mirrors. As we walked by each section of the camp, our view of the detainees was framed by words condemning President Obama, the United States, and our corrupt legal system, asking us as visitors why they were still being held there indefinitely, with no end in sight.

When I asked the commanding officer why they permitted the protest placards, he replied that it "keeps order in the camps" when the detainees feel their voices are heard.

As we exited Camp 6 to pass briefly through Camp 5, modeled after a maximum-security prison, we heard a detainee howling in excruciating pain, calling out to Allah and to the Americans to witness the injustice in the camps. We peered down an adjoining hallway and saw a detainee strapped to a chair, held down by restraints on his arms and legs, being force-fed with the type of nasal G-tube that I had, minutes before, been holding in my hands. He was wailing in a mixture of Arabic and English, but it could easily have been ancient Greek.

His words reverberated down the hallway, echoing like the voice of Prometheus against the Scythian cliffs:

PROMETHEUS
Witness
how the gods
now cause

me to suffer,
inflicting
immeasurable
pain upon one
of their own!

Look upon
the tortures
I shall endure
over this end-
less sentence,
passed by
the newly
self-appointed
patriarch
of the gods,
the so-called
blessed ones!

Listen as
I groan
in misery,
then hear
me moan for
the misery
to come!

Who knows
how long
the suffering
will last, and

when I will
finally be
relieved?

The detainee could not see us. How many times must he have made that speech in the hope that someone from the outside might hear it? But his words would not be heard; nor would they travel beyond the thick, reinforced walls of the detention camps. Like Prometheus, he was calling out for justice. But inside, his words were of little value. It was only through action that his story might reach the outside world.

Although hunger strikes and mass suicide attempts began at Gitmo as early as 2002, the first major hunger strike that was reported in the press took place in 2005, when as many as two hundred detainees refused to eat in protest of the conditions in the camps. The strike ended after twenty-six days, when DOD officials agreed to adhere to the Geneva Conventions. In the years to come, the hunger strikes continued—on and off—sometimes en masse, other times on an individual basis, culminating in a six-month strike in 2013. At its peak, 106 out of 166 detainees stopped consuming food. The strike began, detainees said, when Gitmo staff sacrilegiously searched and mishandled personal copies of the Koran. The military maintained that no desecration of Korans had taken place and that the alleged abuse was an excuse detainees used for staging the strike.

The origins of the 2013 strike are still disputed, but according to a *New York Times* story by Charlie Savage, "both detainee lawyers and military officials agreed that the underlying cause of the protest was the growing despair of the inmates over whether they would ever go home alive." Time and time again a combination of anger and despair had motivated the detainees to use their bodies as weapons. By hurting themselves, they damaged the image and reputation of the country that was keeping them captive. When I asked a rear admiral about tensions with detainees, he told me about a note that one of the men in Camp 5 had sent him: the man vowed that he would leave Guantánamo either on a stretcher or on a gurney. There would be neither submission nor surrender.

In the prologue of *Prometheus Bound,* three gods lead Prometheus to the "end of the earth." Two of them, Kratos and Bia, whose names respectively mean "Power" and "Force," appear to be devoid of all sympathy for Prometheus and carry out their work with almost sadistic pleasure, mocking and abusing him as they imprison him on the cliffs of Scythia. They order the third god, Hephaestus, god of metallurgy and blacksmiths, to nail Prometheus's body to the side of the precipice with his "unbreakable chains." Suddenly overwhelmed with emotion, Hephaestus hesitates to act, whereupon Power and Force admonish him for going soft. Compelled by Power and Force, he then pounds nails through Prometheus's hands and feet and through the center of his chest, causing him profound pain.

As Prometheus howls and writhes in agony, Hephaestus expresses sympathy for the prisoner.

> HEPHAESTUS
> Prometheus.
> I groan with
> you, as if your
> pain were mine.

His companions are quick to castigate him for over-identifying with the prisoner.

> KRATOS
> Be careful
> who you groan
> for, or you
> may end up
> groaning
> yourself.

> HEPHAESTUS
> How can you
> witness his
> pain and not
> avert your eyes?

> KRATOS
> It is easy
> to watch
> him get

what he
deserves.

Aeschylus's choice to portray two types of gods in
the prologue—two devoid of compassion, and one so
overcome with pity and shame that he is unable to carry
out his job—reminded me of something that George
Adkinson had told me about the types of people who
work inside prisons. On the one hand, he said, "you had
your enforcers," tough, sometimes mean-spirited corrections officers who asserted power and used force and
intimidation to keep the prisoners in line. On the other
hand, "you had your patsies, people who were easily
taken advantage of by the inmates." Then "there were
many others who walked the fence. Certain people were
not afraid to get physical with the inmates," but "others
were simply scared of their own shadows."

Most corrections officers were in the third category,
he said, falling somewhere in between, and the truth
of that observation became more than apparent as we
presented scenes from *Prometheus* for corrections staff.
During the discussion following the first performance in
Missouri, a corrections officer standing in the back of
the auditorium launched into a long, loud rant about
how there would be fewer people in prison today if parents were still allowed to corporally punish their children. The man, turning red in the face, spoke forcefully
and angrily. When he was finished, he walked out the
door.

Others that night spoke compassionately, even tenderly, about connections they had made with inmates, reflecting upon the transformations they had witnessed in prison. After the event, a slight woman in a yellow shirt with the weathered look of a chain smoker approached me in tears. Taking my hand, she said, "Thank you for doing this. No one ever thinks to do anything for us. This elevated our profession." Since the performance was voluntarily attended, the crowd was naturally self-selecting, skewing in the direction of those who saw their role as rehabilitative; but as we continued performing in correctional and detention settings, following each performance, the age-old tension between Hephaestus on one side and Power and Force on the other was palpably present in the audiences.

Back at Gitmo, in a packed auditorium in a building adjacent to the main headquarters, the Tony Award–winning Irish actor Brían F. O'Byrne finished his chilling portrayal of Prometheus for a diverse audience of guards, Marines, FBI agents, interpreters, military lawyers, and navy and army officers—including a four-star general and a one-star admiral, both seated in the front row. I then turned to the audience to ask some of the questions I had posed to the corrections officials in Missouri.

The range of answers that came back candidly that day, from all parts of the auditorium, forced me to reevaluate many of my presumptions and judgments about the audience for whom we were performing. Some of the testimonials and unfettered opinions given by audience members about the mission at Gitmo could also have been made by Power and Force, while others spoke with the caution and contrition of Hephaestus.

"Who is Prometheus? Have you ever seen him? Have you worked with him?" I asked.

"I am Prometheus," a guard in the back offered. "I am the one who is chained to this rock—this island—at the end of the earth." He felt isolated in Camp Delta, he said; he couldn't tell his relatives where he was stationed, fearing their judgment, and even within the military there was a stigma associated with working at Gitmo. The guards were isolated from the rest of the world, on the southern tip of Cuba. Heads unanimously nodded in agreement. As the guard spoke his mind, it suddenly struck me that we had been given access to something that very few Americans would ever see or hear, and now it was our job to try to listen empathetically, without judgment, in spite of how difficult it might prove to be.

Most of the guards we met were eighteen to twenty-four years old and had been deployed to Gitmo as a first or second assignment. Some who worked in the maximum-security facilities, such as Camp 5, were military police with years of correctional training under their belts. But many of the rest had been infantry, mortar-men, drivers, or gunners and had received one month of training. They had learned a handful of words in Arabic and Pashto, the Iranian language spoken in Afghanistan, before being thrust into the ethical fog of Guantánamo Bay. Their job was to keep order within the camps, to protect the detainees, and to prevent suicides and assaults. They were never to retaliate against the detainees, their so-called enemies, who in many cases were much more sophisticated—intellectually and psychologically—than they. Many of the detainees would do their best to provoke a reaction, by jeering at them and by celebrating the deaths of their friends, in order to prove their moral superiority.

When the young god Hermes visits Prometheus, at the end of the play, and appeals to him to share what he knows about the downfall and destruction that he has brazenly, vocally predicted for Zeus, Prometheus mocks him, in much the same way I imagined the detainees mocked many of the guards at Gitmo.

PROMETHEUS
Boldly spoken,
and with a lot of heart,
especially for an assistant.

You are so young,
your power so new.

Like some petulant
adolescent you think
your house is made
of unbreakable boards.

But I have
seen the two
before him
plummet

from above,
just as I will
one day see
him plunge
from power,
quickly and
shamefully.

Did you somehow
suppose I would
cringe when you
came, shaking in
the presence of
a god still wet
behind the ears?

Then, I hate to be
the one to tell you,
son, nothing could be
further from the truth.

Run along now.

Hurry back to the one
who sent you here, for
you will learn nothing
from questioning me.

"I work with Prometheus every day," said another
guard, seated in the second-to-last row. He proceeded to

tell a graphic story about an angry detainee who hurled urine and feces into his face and taunted him and his family back home with violent threats. As the attack occurred, he said, a mix of emotions coursed through his mind—a desire to retaliate and a fear that he might not be able to stop himself from retaliating.

While he spoke, a Marine seated in the front of the auditorium, with bulging biceps that seemed like they could, at any minute, rip straight through the tightly rolled sleeves of his desert cammies, noticeably tensed up and turned red, as if steam were about to shoot out from his ears.

When the guard finished his account of the attack, the Marine swiveled around in his seat to address him, as well as the audience. "Thank you for sharing your story," he said, his cheeks still flushed with rage, "but I want you to know that as soon as we get these *enemies* back on enemy soil and back in the crosshairs of our weapons, I assure you, we will have the last laugh." Then, for emphasis, in case someone in the audience had not been listening, or had not understood that he was voicing a desire to kill the very men whom they had sworn to keep alive, he repeated himself: "We will have the last laugh."

For a brief moment, no one said a word, and I let the comment hang in the air in the hope that someone with a different point of view might respond to it.

As the discussion continued, the people who lived and worked at Gitmo seemed to be sharing their deeply conflicted feelings about the mission in an open forum for the first time. Most notably, the presence of the silent four-star general in the front row did not appear to inhibit the conversation. This atmosphere of permissiveness resulting from Aeschylus's ancient play, which seemed to strip away rank and uniform, became most apparent when I asked my final question.

After Prometheus spurns the help of his relatives and friends, drives away his closest allies, taunts Hermes, and openly undermines the authority of Zeus, he provokes the very punishment that has been his objective all along. In his final lines, as Zeus's dark thunderclouds gather on the horizon and begin barreling toward him, you can almost taste his excitement, as well as his terror:

PROMETHEUS
Oh Mother!
Oh Sacred Earth!
Oh Heavenly Sky,
where the sunlight
always shines!

Witness the injustice
of my suffering!

As Brían O'Byrne delivered these lines, I could not help but think about the detainee whom I had witnessed being restrained and force-fed as he cried to Allah, to President Obama, and—most important—to us to witness what was being done to him.

In the final minutes of the discussion, I turned to

the audience to ask the question that had been burning within me since I first set foot in Guantánamo Bay. "At the end of the play, when Zeus punishes Prometheus, who then becomes the most iconic martyr of all time, who wins—"

Down front a Judge Advocate General's Corps (JAG) lawyer rose to his feet, cut me off, and addressed the crowd. "I'm glad you asked that question, because we have lost all moral authority in this war and will never regain it until we give these men fair trials." He went on to describe how frustrating and heartbreaking it had been to watch helplessly as the United States betrayed its own values by indefinitely deferring justice for the detainees.

As a theater director, I often know how an audience is reacting to a performance by the way people are breathing. Sometimes during powerful moments, when actors are able to convey the truth of an experience, audience members begin breathing together, inhaling and exhaling as one. Whenever this happens, the quality of the silence in the theater deepens, and the audience listens with a level of attention that is rarely achieved in today's fast-paced world.

At several points during our multiple performances at Gitmo, over both visits, I sensed this happening. As if to validate my observation, we discovered the following comment by a soldier on an audience feedback form, collected after one of the early showings of Theater of War. "Felt like I could breathe again for the first time." Judging from the way audience members at

Gitmo breathed, watched, and listened, the JAG lawyer was not alone in his moral discomfort. They were all chained to a rock—an island—at the end of the earth, and for a brief moment, as a community, they were all acutely aware of it.

HERACLES IN HOSPICE

I

It is 3:15 a.m. I am hovering over Laura in our East Village apartment, listening to her laboring to breathe, watching her chest rise and fall, and wondering if there is anything I can do to relieve her pain. I've taken a sleeping pill, but there is no way I am sleeping tonight. Snow is piling up in drifts on the unplowed streets outside our loft. The wind howls against the window as if screaming to be let in from the cold. The night nurse rises from her chair in the corner of the open room and administers another dose of morphine, but Laura keeps laboring.

At this point in the progression of her disease and her body's rejection of the foreign organs, the double lung transplant she received not nineteen months ago, to breathe means to suffer. So according to this sinister arithmetic, a precondition of Laura's existence and her remaining time on earth is unrelenting suffering. When she is conscious, her agony is almost too much to witness. It's not something that humans, even with their insatiable appetite for violence and indefatigable ability to inflict pain upon one another, could ever have invented. It's a suffering so creative and cunning, so endlessly innovative and resourceful, that it is beyond human intelligence. Watching Laura suffer is a spiritual experience, because it points to something beyond humanity, a cruelty that can only be divine.

When she drifts off to sleep, all I can do is hope that she will never wake again. The night nurse, standing at my side, looks over at me with knowing, penetrating eyes, as if she has stood in this very spot before, in this very apartment, at 3:15 in the morning, reading my mind. Then she administers a second dose of morphine. Then, minutes later, another. I do nothing to stop her. In fact, a part of me is praying that the morphine will depress Laura's respiratory system, once and for all, and put her out of her misery. Another part of me is wondering if my wish for Laura to die is simply the result of my own limitations, my weakness, my inability to stand by and see things to their natural conclusion. By standing here silently as the nurse administers more and more medication, will my hands be stained with her blood? Will I be hounded by this memory for the rest of my life? Am I a murderer? These are the thoughts coursing through my emotionally exhausted, sleep-deprived brain.

Laura's breathing slows. Her chest no longer rises and falls in predictable intervals. Her breaths are shallow now, and slightly erratic. The air remains in the hollow of her neck, barely entering her chest. At some moments, I am not sure if she is breathing at all. Is the ambient light from the lamps in the alley, reflecting off the falling snow, playing tricks on me? I crawl into the bed, curl up in a ball by her side, and drift off into half-consciousness, a kind of light-twilight slumber from which I can easily be aroused, if needed, to administer medication or oxygen at a moment's notice. There will be no dreaming tonight, no losing myself in the sub-conscious abyss, in spite of the little blue pill I ingested hours earlier. I am resting my eyes, or so I tell myself, at the moment when sleep finally comes, stealing me away to dreamland.

When I awaken the next morning to a pile of fresh snow stacked on the windowsill, I half-expect to turn over and find a cold blue corpse resting next to me. Part of me wishes it were so. But there she is, laboring and awake. Her skeletal frame has grown so tolerant of the opiates we have been pumping into her veins that no amount of morphine will ever relieve her suffering. Worst of all, I have no way to explain to her the thousand contradictory thoughts racing through my mind, no words to convey how sorry I am that she is still alive, and how relieved I am to wake and find her still breathing there beside me.

At the end of *Women of Trachis,* Sophocles's most over-looked and underestimated play, is a scene that speaks to the ethics and emotions surrounding death and dying with timeless power: a man in the throes of unimaginable pain asks his teenage son to help him die. The son at first refuses, and a high-stakes struggle plays out, in which the man threatens to disown his son if the boy doesn't fulfill his dying wish to be burned alive.

The dying man is no ordinary mortal. He is Heracles, a Greek hero who in his life constantly pushed beyond the boundaries of what it means to be human. As the half-mortal son of Alcmene and Zeus, he developed divine aspirations at an early age. A prophecy had foretold that he might one day become a god, so he spent his life attempting to fulfill it through death-defying acts, or "labors," such as slaying a nine-headed Hydra, wrestling the Nemean lion, and capturing Cerberus, the fierce, three-headed hellhound that guards the entrance to Hades. (Later, in Roman mythology, Heracles would be called Hercules.)

In Sophocles's version of the story, when death finally comes for Heracles, it catches him off guard. He had expected one day to be taken down by a mighty adversary in the heat of battle. Instead, his jealous wife, Deianeira, accidentally poisons him with what she believes to be a love potion, distilled from the blood of a centaur. Years earlier, when the centaur attempted to abscond with his young wife, Heracles had shot him with his invincible bow. While gasping his last breaths, the centaur gave Deianeira a vial of his blood, telling her it possessed the power to make Heracles love her again, after her radiant beauty began to fade. (Lesson number one: never trust a dying centaur.)

At the beginning of Sophocles's play, Heracles returns from one of his recent conquests with a stunning young war bride, Iole. After laying eyes on the girl, Deianeira immediately sends her husband a robe soaked in the centaur's blood, desperately hoping to regain his affection. Heracles gladly accepts the welcoming gesture and triumphantly slips the robe over his broad shoulders. But as soon as sunlight touches the fabric, the poisoned garment brings him to his knees as it eats straight through his flesh, tearing through ligaments and tendons, liquefying his muscles and bones. Howling in agony, he calls for his soldiers to put him out of his misery.

HERACLES
It has me in its teeth.
Ahhhhhhhhhhhhhhh!
It feeds on me again.
Ahhhhhhhhhhhhhhh!

Where are you from?
You call yourself "Greeks"?

You are the most
unrighteous, unjust,
unworthy of men.

I wore myself
down to the bone
for you so-called
Greeks, ridding
your country of
monsters and

exterminating
sea beasts.

Now that I am
the one moaning
on the ground,
clutching my
sides in pain,
will one of you
please come
quickly and visit
me with a sword
or a torch?

Heracles's once-great arms, which defeated the most fearsome of beasts, are no longer strong enough to lift his body from the ground. But true to form, he summons what little energy remains and attempts to take charge of his final moments on earth. He wishes to die a great death, one that will live on in legend for all time. So he calls his teenage son, Hyllus, to his side and asks for assistance. He grabs Hyllus's hand and forces him to swear an oath to carry his body to the top of Oeta, the sacred mountain of Zeus, and set it on fire.

HYLLUS
Father, what
are you saying?

What are you
asking me to do?

HERACLES
What must
be done. Or
be someone
else's son!

HYLLUS
I ask you again,
Father, what are
you asking me
to do—be your
murderer, stained
with the pollution
of your blood,
and hounded by
Furies forever?

HERACLES
I am asking you
to be my doctor.
Heal this affliction!
Cure my disease!

For some people today, attempting to exert control over the process of dying could mean taking narcotics, while refusing food and water, and slipping quietly away into blissful, endless sleep. For the great Greek hero, it meant going out in a blaze of flames. So Heracles commands his son to be his "doctor" by burning him alive in a ritual, atop Mount Oeta, aimed at cementing his status as the immortal son of Zeus. Some scholars have argued that at the end of Sophocles's play, Heracles transforms into a god in a moment of ascension, or apotheosis. Others contend that he simply dies. Though nothing in the surviving script resolves this question, one thing is certain: Heracles knew how to make a dramatic exit, one that would be remembered for many centuries to come.

The word that Heracles uses for doctor—*iater,* "one who heals" or "physician"—would have had special resonance when *Women of Trachis* was first performed. During this period, medicine—ranging from drugs and surgery to salves and incantations—straddled the line between a spiritual and a scientific discipline. Doctors and other types of healers proliferated throughout Greece, while cults worshipping Asclepius, the god of medicine and healing, developed and spread over a wide geographic area. Around 420 BC a prominent temple to Asclepius—or clinic—was established in Athens, on the south slope of the Acropolis, next to the Theater of Dionysus. It was one of the primary care facilities in Athens during the late fifth century BC.

Sick suppliants would approach such temples, kneel before the priests of Asclepius, bow their heads, and ask to be healed. They would pray and make sacrifices and would be instructed to sleep in the temple—or *asklepeion*—where the god would visit them in dreams, sometimes in the form of a snake. He would treat the patients as they slept, healing them in dreams. The next morning patients would report their dreams to the priests and would be prescribed additional remedies.

I once stood in the ruins of the Temple of Asclepius in Athens at dusk. Next door, standing on the far side of the Theater of Dionysus, a female docent was speaking in Modern Greek in hushed tones into her cell phone. I could hear her words with near-perfect clarity, as if listening to noise-canceling headphones. In ancient times, I was sure, anyone who visited the Temple of Asclepius would have been able to hear the plays of Sophocles and other ancient poets being performed in the adjacent theater with more clarity than I heard that docent. In other words, the theater and the clinic were somehow interconnected.

One classical scholar, Robin Mitchell-Boyask, has asserted a direct therapeutic link between the Theater of Dionysus and the Temple of Asclepius, not just in Athens but throughout the Hellenic world. Healing temples were often placed in proximity to amphitheaters, he argues, for a medical reason. "Given the Greek belief in the healing powers of song," he states in the medical journal *The Lancet*, "this placement was not coincidental."

The Greek word for "healing song," *paean*, also referred to a song of praise for the god Apollo. Through songs of prayer, suppliants were healed. In the Homeric epics, the physician of the gods was named Paean. A *paean*, one might argue, was the most common form of medicine—the antibiotic of the ancient Greek world. Menander, a Greek dramatist of the fourth century BC, wrote that "language is the healer of the soul." The word for *theater* in Greek, *theatron*, means "the seeing place," but perhaps it was actually the "hearing place," where citizens and foreigners went to listen to the healing songs and words of the tragic poets. In the Theater of Dionysus, the highly stylized costumes, masks, and movements of Greek tragedy provided a visual spectacle, but audience members sitting in the back would likely have heard more of the play than they saw.

But what was healing or helpful about hearing suffering characters scream in pain?

Between 430 and 426 BC, according to the ancient historian Thucydides, a virulent plague wiped out nearly 30 percent of the Athenian population. During those same few years, Athens suffered catastrophic losses in a freshly launched war with its neighbor, Sparta. Given the extenuating circumstances during this period, it seems natural that Athenians might have gone to the theater in search of comfort, if not relief from what ailed them. But if tragedy served a therapeutic function in Athenian society, how did it work, beyond Aristotle's enigmatic concept of catharsis as the cleansing of pity and fear?

Perhaps the Athenian appetite for the type of unbridled anguish, grief, and trauma depicted on stage by Sophocles and his contemporaries grew from a need to give voice to the widespread, pervasive suffering that many Athenians had experienced firsthand—during the plague and over a century of perpetual military conflict.

After all, between the Athenian plague and the Peloponnesian War, almost everyone in the audience would have personally witnessed or experienced the kind of physical pain and existential anguish portrayed in Greek tragedy.

The most famous and best-regarded tragedy to survive the ancient world, Sophocles's *Oedipus the King,* debuted in Athens in 429 BC, the year after the plague first struck the city. Not surprisingly, it directly references and describes the Athenian plague in graphic detail, except that the play is set in archaic Thebes. As the tragedy begins, a group of sickly Theban elders appear on their knees before the palace to ask King Oedipus to heal the city.

> PRIEST
> A savage pestilence
> has ravaged the land,
> killing the cattle
> and the crops.
>
> Our women
> die in labor,
> delivering
> shriveled
> little corpses,
> as the hateful
> plague spreads
> like a raging
> wildfire,

devouring
the city without
mercy, emptying
homes, and
filling the streets
with moans and
wailing and heaps
of rotting bodies,
while death-rich
Hades makes off
with the shades.

Why did Sophocles go to such lengths to describe the Athenian plague, but set it in archaic Thebes? Passages such as the one above point toward a way not just of interpreting tragedy but of using it to help people confront the most pressing challenges of their day.

Greek tragedy, it seems, permits audiences to look at the present moment through the lens of the distant mythological past, in order to see more clearly what cannot be perceived up close, affording a healthier perspective, a longer view. Also, by creating a forum for citizens and foreigners to come together, to acknowledge what they've been through, and to collectively share their pain and suffering, the tragic poets—in a sense—may have been the de facto healers of the polis, dispensing their medicine, as Michell-Boyask suggests, right next to the clinic, in the center of Athens.

II

All the boy wanted, his entire life, was to be loved by his father. And by loved, he really meant accepted, though he didn't know how to say it. He wished to hear the words "Well done, son," while being slapped on the back, or having his neck forcefully kneaded by a muscular hand, after doing something that had awakened his father's pride. In fact, simply hearing the word *son*, spoken tenderly and with a modicum of affection, would have endowed him with far more security and self-assurance in the world than he currently possessed.

His famous father had been away, either at war or attempting one of many superhuman exploits, for nearly all his childhood. Truthfully, he did not know him. What little he did know about him, he had pieced together from offhand comments made by his mother when she had imbibed too much wine, or from rumor or legend, which, when it came to Heracles, always seemed to be in abundance. Like the legend of how Heracles had burned an entire city to the ground on behalf of some princess he wished to wed. Heracles never accepted no for an answer. If he wanted something, especially something he felt he was due, he would take it. So even if the story was unsubstantiated, the boy knew in his heart that it was something his father would do. Though perhaps factually untrue, it conveyed something truthful about Heracles.

Now that Hyllus was on the verge of becoming a man, and would soon be taking on all the responsibilities of the title, he needed to know—now more than ever—that Heracles cared about him, even in absentia. Maybe he was too sensitive, he often thought, slapping his forehead repeatedly with the palm of his hand. Perhaps he should have worked harder at cultivating the kind of cold-hearted indifference with which his father had always regarded him. But on that fateful afternoon when he delivered his mother's gift—the stunning purple robe—to welcome his father home as he triumphantly returned from his latest conquest, his entire being yearned for the smallest sign of fondness. For a fleeting moment, he finally received it.

As Heracles stretched out his arms, draping the robe regally over his chest and shoulders, and looking directly at his adolescent son, whom he hadn't seen in more than a year, he smiled. It lasted but a few seconds, before the sunlight hit the robe, unleashing the savage poison of the centaur's blood hiding in its fibers. But the smile spoke volumes, and—perhaps for the first time in his life—Hyllus felt the warmth of his father's love radiating through his veins, like an antidote to his poisonous childhood.

During the fifth century BC, while the cult of Asclepius and other healing sects steadily grew in popularity, the founder of Western medicine, Hippocrates (b. 460 BC), and his followers codified a series of treatises on medicine that still inform the way doctors practice today. The voluminous body of writing generated by these early physicians was aimed at establishing the objectives of medicine, as well as its limits. According to the Hippocratic treatise *On the Art of Medicine,* the medical profession sought to "do away with the sufferings of the sick, to lessen the violence of their diseases, and to refuse to treat those who are overmastered by their disease, realizing that in such cases medicine is powerless."

Since fifth-century-BC Athens had no accreditation process, let alone medical school, just about anyone could claim to be a doctor. In light of the softness of their science, many Hippocratic physicians turned away patients who, in their opinion, were beyond the reach of medicine, presumably in order to protect the legitimacy of the profession and perhaps, as one doctor suggested to me recently, to lower their mortality rates. The practitioners of Hippocratic medicine—unlike many other healers of the time—did not claim to be able to treat or cure all illnesses. However, in refusing to administer to patients who were dying from untreatable conditions, they, in effect, may have hastened patients' deaths or, even worse, prolonged their suffering.

In addition to refusing to treat the terminally ill, another prominent feature of Hippocratic medicine— one that, strikingly, is still upheld by doctors today— was the prohibition of doctor-assisted death. Hippocratic physicians were forbidden to administer "deadly drugs" to anyone if asked, or to recommend such drugs to a suffering patient. This is notable for a number of reasons. Mercy killing, or helping people who were suffering to die, was certainly not illegal in fifth-century-BC Greece; nor was it necessarily taboo. Also, the Greeks had a different relationship to suicide from what we in the West have today, where suicide is seen—often through the lens of Christianity—as a shameful act. Though many disapproved of it, the Greeks did not uniformly see it as a moral failing to take one's own life. In certain instances, they viewed it as acceptable, such as when a person was in prolonged agony; they could even regard it as heroic, as in the famous state-mandated suicide of Socrates.

Perhaps the doctors who wrote the Hippocratic treatises prohibiting physicians from dispensing toxic drugs sought to define medicine as preserving life rather than hastening death. Just as they turned away patients who were beyond treatment, they turned away suffering patients and refused to help them end their lives. Maybe it was a reactionary measure, at a time with little or no professional standards, to preserve the integrity of their school of medical practice?

For these ancient physicians, to reject the sick and to refuse to help suffering patients die was certainly no small gesture, especially given that a vast number of people would have been suffering from ailments far beyond the scope of ancient medicine, such as the plague of 430 BC. Perhaps this is why Sophocles—who was rumored, apocryphally, to have been a priest of Asclepius, and who was said to have kept the god's sacred snake in his home while the Temple of Asclepius was under construction in Athens—chose to explore the ethics and emotions surrounding end-of-life care in such clear relief in the final scene of his *Women of Trachis*.

No one can question that Heracles makes a forceful argument for assisted death in *Women of Trachis*. But Sophocles always worked hard to portray all sides of a struggle with equal weight and sympathy. In the play's final scene, he illuminated the needs and desires of a dying man as forcefully as he depicted the internal conflict of his primary caregiver, Hyllus, contrasting Heracles's anguish and misery with his son's psychological distress.

After agreeing to take his father to Mount Oeta and help burn him alive, Hyllus hesitates, and Heracles unfairly condemns him for it.

> HERACLES
> It seems this boy
> has no intention
> of doing what his
> dying father has
> asked of him!
>
> Know this, son.
>
> You will be cursed
> by the gods if you
> do not give me what
> I am rightfully due.
>
> HYLLUS
> Your words will soon betray
> how sick you really are.

HERACLES
Yes, for you have
enraged the pain,
awakening it again.

HYLLUS
This is impossible.
No matter what
I decide to do,
I will be wrong.

HERACLES
Yes, because you
think it is right
to disobey a father.

HYLLUS
If I am loyal
to you, then
I am disloyal
to myself and
my sense of
what is right.

Is this the lesson
that I am to learn?

HERACLES
You will learn
the meaning
of loyalty

by granting
happiness to
a dying man.

Hyllus strongly voices his distress at being asked to
do something that violates his own moral compass. His
fear of betraying his father through inaction is matched
by a fear of betraying himself and his values, by doing
something that he will likely regret for the rest of his
life. Hyllus will either wrong his father or be wronged
by him, and this conflict exemplifies the very essence of
Greek tragedy. Sophocles's tragedies, in particular, all
seem to depict a universe in which passionate people
with mutually opposed desires and visions of the world
struggle to do what they believe is justified or correct,
but ultimately—regardless of what they decide to do—
will be wrong.

Deciding to help or to refuse to help someone who
is suffering to die is one of the most ethically complex
decisions a human being can make, and Hyllus, in spite
of his relative youth, navigates the situation as gracefully as possible, carving out his own indemnity, by limiting his role in his father's death. He builds the pyre
but does not light it, and most important, he reconfirms
Heracles's wishes—out in the open—for everyone to
hear.

HYLLUS
Then you order
me to do this
with full under-

standing of what
you are saying?

HERACLES
Yes, I call out
to the gods
to bear witness
to my words.

HYLLUS
Since you have
shown these deeds
to the gods to be
yours, not mine,
then I will do what
you have asked,
and then no one
will ever be able to
question my loyalty.

HERACLES
In the end,
you have
chosen well,
my son.

The public nature of Hyllus's struggle to protect himself and his own interests while helping his father to die is integral to the power of Sophocles's play and its impact upon audiences. In a 1985 article in the *Archives of Internal Medicine,* entitled "Limiting Treatment in a Social Vacuum: A Greek Chorus for William T.," the bioethicist Kathryn Montgomery Hunter argues that the ethical insight of Greek tragedy resides not just in its content but in its form and, in particular, in the chorus.

The convention of the chorus has baffled and mystified audiences, as well as directors, for centuries. At best, choruses seem to state the obvious and repeat arguments that have already been made on stage by the primary characters; rarely do they play a role in instigating or resolving the conflict. However, according to Hunter, the chorus—as proxy for the audience watching the play—provides a communal model or framework for distributing the burden of complex ethical and legal decisions evenly upon a group of active witnesses and participants, rather than solely upon an individual. The chorus, Hunter writes, plays a crucial role in the protagonist's struggle, through its "presence and its sympathy and its clear meditation on his or her predicament in a social and historical context." Most important, the chorus ensures that the characters are almost never alone on stage. A community of stakeholders is always present.

The chorus in *Women of Trachis* is a group of local women, servants of Heracles's wife, Deianeira. When they first hear that Heracles's limp, lifeless body is being carried toward them on the shoulders of his soldiers, they collectively grieve and agonize over his fate. In their struggle to understand what has become of Heracles, we hear the sympathy and concern of a community as it responds to the suffering of an individual. The chorus remains silent for most of the final scene, but its presence is always felt, as Hyllus and Heracles wrestle with their complex predicament.

One of the chief problems for families and physicians faced with the task of making end-of-life decisions on behalf of incapacitated patients, who—unlike Heracles—have not made their wishes known through an advanced directive, is that they usually must make them in isolation rather than in the presence of a community of stakeholders—such as friends, family members, and medical professionals. Sadly, they must decide in a "social vacuum" in which the patient's personal history cannot fully be represented or known; the specific legal and medical arguments for and against a course of action are not vigorously explored or debated. Left to make end-of-life decisions on their own, individuals are burdened with their full moral and spiritual weight. Many people in this position, no matter what decision they make, understandably end up feeling like Hyllus, responsible either for prolonging the person's suffering or for bringing about death, "stained with the pollution" of an impossible decision.

The tragic chorus, in addition to being a poetic form, is a highly rhetorical form, characterized by *strophes* and *antistrophes*—in Greek, "turning" and "turning back." These words denote the synchronized left-right dance of two sections of the chorus as they move from one side of the orchestra to the other; the words also describe the opposing arguments that the divided chorus makes as it struggles with the issues presented in the play. The job of the chorus in a Greek tragedy, according to Hunter, is "to present the conflict, agonize over its consequences for the hero and for the community," and "reflect on its history and its moral significance." In other words, it bears witness to the tragic events unfolding and worries about their potential consequences.

When Hyllus asks his father to "order" him to carry out his final wishes, he is attempting to spread the ethical burden of Heracles's death upon all those present who hear his words. The chorus watches and remembers. It listens and records. Its silent presence ensures that Hyllus does not have to act alone and be "stained with his father's blood." It hears Heracles's order and participates in helping the suffering hero die.

The chorus is the opposite of a social vacuum. In fact, when Hyllus finally brings Heracles to Mount Oeta to die, Heracles rides, quite literally, upon the shoulders of the community.

> HYLLUS
> Hoist him upon your
> shoulders, friends,
> showing compassion
> for what has happened,
> witnessing the brutality
> of the gods toward
> one they called a son.
>
> No one can say
> what is to come.

It is heartbreaking
to helplessly look
upon this man's
suffering, and
shameful for those
who cause it, but
hardest of all upon
the one who suffers
this affliction.

Women of Trachis concludes with a profound vision for how to face death. Instead of abandoning the terminally ill, or declining to treat them, or refusing to help them die in accordance with their wishes, the community must gather around the patient and his family to listen, agonize, debate, and—ultimately—carry on their shoulders the burden of whatever must be done.

III

As Theater of War continued to tour, new projects naturally evolved out of our work with the military that were designed to address the needs of other communities. One of these projects, End of Life, presents readings of scenes from Sophocles's *Women of Trachis* and *Philoctetes* in medical settings as a catalyst for open dialogue about the ethics and emotions of end-of-life care. After one such reading at Harvard Medical School for an audience of students and medical professionals, a male hospice nurse with long white hair, wearing a faded jean jacket, approached a microphone in the center of one of the auditorium aisles.

His hands trembling, he nervously said, "Forgive me. I've never spoken before in public in my entire life. . . . But I feel compelled to apologize to all of the doctors in the audience who do not get to be with their patients when they die. I have a hard job. But I witness miracles every day."

The nurse had no intention of glamorizing death or dying. His point was simply that there is more to medicine than preserving life, and that doctors who no longer interact with patients when they are deemed beyond treatment are deprived of experiencing an integral part of life, namely death.

Later that summer, after another performance at Harvard, this time for an ethics course, a senior oncologist on the verge of tears quietly told a crowd of friends and colleagues: "I have never—in all my years of practicing medicine—questioned my position on euthanasia until hearing the screams of the actor playing Heracles tonight."

Doctors are trained in the West to practice their craft with detachment. This makes practical sense, as they must witness suffering every day. Starting in medical school, they build up walls to protect themselves from unwanted emotions. And so I hoped a performance of extreme suffering—such as in Sophocles's depiction of Heracles's death—might touch doctors and other health professionals in unexpected ways, opening up dialogue about the challenges of witnessing suffering.

My own experiences as a caregiver taught me that death is an opportunity—just like birth—for generating deeper levels of connection between people and vivid memories that can last a lifetime. When we confront the death of someone we love, as Hyllus does for Heracles in *Women of Trachis,* we must discover—on our own terms—how best to help the dying person while simultaneously protecting ourselves and our own interests. This is by no means easy, even for those with years of experience. By relegating dialogue about death and dying either to closeted conversations between patients, family members, and doctors or to shouting matches between politically opposed factions, we are, as a culture, depriving ourselves of the ability to talk openly about a serious challenge that all of us will likely one day face.

The hospice and palliative care professionals who visited our apartment during the last months of Laura's life were among the noblest, wisest people I have ever met. They are the unsung heroes of modern medicine and largely work on its margins. With sensitivity and compassion, they guided us through difficult moments with steady assurance and encouraged us to take risks, at critical junctures when maintaining Laura's quality of life was more important than her living. Had these fine individuals not been quietly present in our apartment during the darkest moments, when Laura was consumed by overwhelming panic or pain, calling out for an end to her suffering, I am not sure I would have survived the intense three-month period between when she checked out of the hospital for the last time and when she died.

By bringing the End of Life project to Harvard Medical School, I hoped to empower hospice and palliative care professionals and other caregivers to come out of the shadows and speak the truth of their experiences, to create a forum where their unique voices and perspectives could be heard. When the hospice nurse spoke after the first performance, I knew the project had the potential to create the conditions for a conversation that many people wanted but few knew how to start: an open discussion of death and dying framed by empathy and experience. As my theater company, Outside the Wire, began to tour with the play, one of the most striking and insightful medical professionals to step out of the shadows was a palliative care doctor at the University of Virginia Medical Center named Leslie Blackhall.

Dr. Blackhall credits her father's death, when she was in third grade, as the reason she went to medical school. He had leukemia, and for a year he had been dying slowly, agonizingly, in front of her. She remembers, at age eight, becoming acutely aware of human mortality, which led her to ask questions that few third graders typically contemplate. Witnessing her father die, and caring for him through his final months, left her "with this burning sense that life is short. And if life is short, then what are we supposed to do with it? If anyone can die, it can't just be to grow up and get a job at GE, which is why my father lived in Schenectady, and then settle down."

As fate would have it, Blackhall ended up studying medicine in New York City during the height of the AIDS epidemic, when little was known about the disease and few precautions were in place. Not until her third-year medical rotation did doctors discover they were dealing with an infectious disease. Up until that point, she remembers "drawing everybody's blood with no gloves." Bellevue Hospital, where she worked, was filled with "young, terribly suffering, dying men." She and her colleagues felt helpless in the face of this modern plague, as it ravaged the city's gay population.

She started to question what it meant to be a doctor when all her patients were going to die. "I mean, if your goal is to cure everybody, then you are a hundred percent going to be failing, over the long run. So how do you become a doctor for mortals?" Unfortunately, the national discussion about the legal and ethical issues surrounding end-of-life care was still new. None of her instructors were teaching how to administer medicine for the dying. The directive was to preserve life at all costs.

Then Blackhall had an experience that fundamentally changed her relationship to medicine and to death. On her first day working as a medical student at New York University Hospital, a resident brought her into a room to see a patient. The woman "had an NG tube in, a nasal gastric tube. She must have had bowel obstruction, because black stuff was pouring out of it. She's writhing there in the bed. Her family is standing around her, and they're dabbing her forehead with a cloth because they didn't know what else to do. We walked in, looked. Then we walked out and closed the door. The resident turned to me and said, 'She'll be dead tonight.' And she was by the next morning."

What haunted Blackhall about the suffering woman was that "nobody lent a helping hand, nobody." From the hospital's perspective, the patient was beyond the scope of medical care, and so its physicians had no business lingering in her room or offering to help ease her suffering. Blackhall awoke that day to the stark reality that doctors did not treat death and dying as a normal part of medicine, and she made it her personal mission to see that they one day would.

Not long afterward, while Blackhall was working the night shift at the hospital, she encountered a patient who was shaking uncontrollably from fever and chills. All he wanted was a blanket, but like the woman in her previous story, he had been left to die in his room, ostensibly without medical care. She went and got him a blanket, even though he wasn't her patient. The man was so touched by this gesture that he teared up and said, "Oh my God, you're an angel." And in that simple exchange, when a doctor attended to a dying man by giving him the thing he needed most, Blackhall discovered what she now refers to as her "calling."

Looking back on it all, Blackhall connects witnessing her father's death, and the suffering that led up to it, with her choice to specialize in palliative medicine, which aims at relieving and managing the pain and symptoms associated with serious illnesses. Blackhall had been comfortable talking about death from a very early age. For her entire life, she has believed that dying is a part of living, so she isn't afraid of death. She is able to "go into those rooms and be there with people. Just be there. And somehow that was really helpful and really important, being a witness, even if all it took was to get the guy a blanket."

In Sophocles's *Women of Trachis,* when Heracles asks his son to be his doctor, his *iater,* he is not asking for medicine. Dehumanized by his condition, he is asking for his son to take his needs seriously and treat him like a human. From Blackhall's perspective, "It's not just about whether it's ethical to do *x* or *y*. It's also about taking care of that lady in the room with the black liquid pouring out of her NG tube and the family dabbing her forehead. It's one thing to say she should have been able to have an assisted suicide. But you know what? She did not have to be suffering that much. Knowing what I know now, her family didn't have to be dabbing her. She didn't have to be writhing in pain. It wasn't just bad ethics, it was crappy medical care."

However one feels about assisted suicide, Blackhall contends, people should not have to choose between agonizing pain and death. It's a false choice, one that is ethically bankrupt from the start. The verb *palliate,* derived from the Latin *palliare,* "to conceal or cloak," means "to alleviate the symptoms of serious, life-threatening illness." Although palliative care still exists on the margins of medical practice, the movement supporting it has gained momentum over the past few decades, since Blackhall began her studies. Moreover, the definition of who gets palliative care and when has been expanded beyond gravely ill patients on the brink of death to patients living with chronic, long-term conditions, struggling to maintain dignity and quality of life.

Fortunately, Blackhall's voice is no longer alone in the wilderness. She now belongs to a growing chorus of medical professionals who see palliative medicine as a serious discipline that should be integral to mainstream training and practice.

Still, the forces in our culture working against the palliative care and hospice movements remain strong, driven by a pervasive fear of death. After decades of caring for the sick and dying, Blackhall has concluded that one of the main reasons our society is so death-averse is that contemplating our own mortality forces us to face profoundly disruptive questions about who we are, our beliefs, and the way we've lived our lives.

I think we all have to acknowledge that dying, the moment of death, is always going to be fearful and mysterious. And no matter how much you believe in an afterlife, or in rebirth, or the peace of the grave, everybody dies. And it's okay that it happens. But there is no way that death isn't going to rupture your reality. And that calls into question what it means to be you. So if doctors, nurses, chaplains, patients, family members, social workers, could face that, we'd be better off. What does it mean for all of us to be mortal? And what does it mean to be a doctor when everyone's mortal? Facing those questions is not necessarily comfortable.

When Blackhall contemplates her own age—fifty-seven—and thinks about the inevitability of death, she is galvanized to make her time on this earth matter. Death helps her to keep her life in focus, to dispense with the things that do not matter and concentrate on what she cares about most. Each person, she holds, must find a way to face death and be present in the face of dying. Her way is to cultivate and maintain a vigilant appreciation of the time she has left, and to help others do the same—through a lust for life, through humor, and through an ability to laugh and find joy in the face of what others might view as a tragedy.

On one home visit to a patient, a painter who was dying of cancer, Blackhall found the man sitting on his bed struggling to do his taxes. He was exhausted and couldn't make sense of the papers spread out around him. "Can you do something about my fatigue?" he asked her. "I'm so tired all the time. Can you help with that?"

And she said, "Well, I might be able to help it a little bit with some medication, but you have to think about how you want to spend the energy you have."

She looked over at the man's son, who had come

home to take care of his father, then back at the man. "I don't think you need to waste your time doing your taxes. I bet someone else could help you do them. But if it's taking all your energy just to do your taxes, and you have only a certain amount of energy, what are you going to do with that energy?"

The man instantly agreed. Then he rose and led her into his studio to show her an unfinished painting, which had been penciled in but not yet painted. It was a commission from a patron.

"How long would it take you to finish something like that in your usual state of health?" she asked.

"Six months," he replied.

The two of them looked at each other. She saw that he lacked the stamina or energy to finish the painting. So she said, "You know, if I was the person who commissioned that, I would appreciate it being framed just the way it is, and to know it was the last thing you did."

The next time she visited the painter, he was sitting on his bed with his family. They were laughing and telling stories. And it was clearly what he needed to be doing. Rather than finish his painting, the man had decided to expend what was left of his energy opening his heart to his family and spending time with them. What mattered most was not doing his taxes, or frantically trying to finish a painting he was never going to complete. What mattered most was being present with those he loved and remembering the wonderful things they had lived through and done together.

As I listened to Blackhall tell this story, it struck me

that the final scene of Sophocles's *Women of Trachis* is painful to witness not just because of the agony of Heracles, as he writhes in pain, screaming in the dirt, but also because of the agony of Hyllus, who so desperately wants to connect with his father and is silently crying out for his affection. The scene almost demands the type of intervention Blackhall described with the painter. Heracles has a finite amount of time left. He can spend it preoccupied by things that are out of his control, or he can spend it bonding with his boy. The tragedy is that, without a true healer to help him see what's most important, he misses out on the opportunity presented by his impending death.

While some people are able to gain important perspective and make powerful connections as they approach death, Blackhall is quick to point out, "some people can't do that. And some people don't want it." When her own mother was dying at home in hospice, Blackhall visited her, but her mother didn't want to think or talk about anything—"she was not a touchy-feely person." Instead, Blackhall would climb into the hospital bed with her mother and silently watch TV with her. Her exhausted mother would rest her head in her lap. "That's how I would touch her. All we did was watch *Home and Garden,* this show in which people got three offers to fix up their den. She loved to watch it. It was a way of distracting her from having to think about the fact that she was dying. It allowed us to sit there together.

"And I still remember the feeling of it. It was snow-ing outside. There was this quality of the light reflecting off the snow. And my mother, who you could never hug, would have her head in my lap because there was no room otherwise for me to watch TV. And I could have my arm on her body, and she could allow that to happen without it really being about how she needed me to hold her. That was as much as she could do. It was one of my best memories of those times."

Some people cannot allow others to be close to them when they die, Blackhall explains. All you can do, if you love them, is try to be present and share moments together. You can't expect people to change that much, just because they're dying—"people are who they are."

The final scene of *Women of Trachis,* in which a father asks his son to end his suffering by ending his life, reminds Blackhall of all the family members she has worked with, over the years, who were led to believe that they were somehow responsible for increasing their loved one's suffering or, worse, had murdered him or her by administering or withholding medication. When Hyllus faces the impossible choice of assisting his father's suicide or being haunted by guilt for not easing his suffering, he cries out, "This is impossible. No matter what I decide to do I will be wrong." Many family members, when facing similarly impossible decisions—such as when to take a patient off a ventilator, remove a feeding tube, or stop medical treatment—feel as if they are living through a Greek tragedy, and that no matter what decision they make, they will be blamed for some moral failing and will have to live with that guilt the rest of their lives. In the end, as with Hyllus, family members feel that their loved one's suffering and death are somehow their fault.

Blackhall is adamant that doctors should work harder to relieve people of this unfair burden. "At the end of life people are demented—they don't swallow, they aspirate, you know. The tubes that you put in somebody's stomach don't work. Families are left to make the decision to forgo hospitalization. And for them, it's like they made the decision to let the patient die.

"I'm sorry, but they're not letting the patient die. The patient is *dying*. If we could heal them, we would. But families are made to feel somehow they're choosing death, or that patients are choosing to die.

"There are studies that say that many family members who make a decision to withdraw medical care in ICU have post-traumatic stress disorder, because it's presented to them as if they were letting their loved one die. You know what? If the doctors thought they could save the patient, they would fight you tooth and nail before they let you withdraw medical care from them. The reason they are talking to you about it is that they think the person is dying. Why can't we convey that adequately in this world?"

This is perhaps the question that motivates Blackhall the most. It's why she gets up in the morning and goes back to the hospital to face death every day.

IV

As End of Life began to tour medical institutions, including Brigham and Women's Hospital, the Cambridge Health Alliance, the University of Virginia Medical Center, and St. Louis Children's Hospital, we started to receive calls from people who had either heard or read about the performances.

In the spring of 2011, a small community hospital in Falmouth, Massachusetts, asked us if we ever presented performances in public. The Falmouth Cancer Committee in collaboration with the Falmouth Public Library wished to host a performance that summer on the town square, on the lawn in front of the library, with the hope of generating much-needed dialogue in the community about end-of-life care.

The town of Falmouth, which has a very large elderly population, was the perfect place to take the project public. The involvement of the cancer committee also seemed fitting, since among medical professionals, oncologists are widely held to be the worst at discussing death with their patients, given their preference for pursuing treatments that extend life by weeks or months. Our project seemed an innovative way to engage the aging population of Falmouth in crucial discussions about end-of-life care. We agreed on July 19 as the performance date and worked with the hospital and library to organize the event, hoping to maximize its reach and impact, with several months of lead time, by getting the word out to a large portion of the local population.

Everything proceeded smoothly and efficiently at first. The hospital committee placed notices in all the Cape Cod cultural calendars, and a local celebrity named Jeff Zinn, artistic director of the Wellfleet Harbor Actors Theater and son of activist writer Howard Zinn, joined the cast. When news traveled that he would be taking part, the town began to buzz with interest and anticipation.

But about two weeks before the performance, I received a call from a woman who worked in the hospital's public relations department, and all the positive momentum came screeching to a sudden halt.

The hospital's ethics committee had decided that it no longer wanted us to perform the final scene from *Women of Trachis* on the town square that July. The caller cited a number of reasons, including the public nature of the performance and the amount of sustained screaming called for in the script. Also, it seemed, the play's explicit depiction of assisted suicide had suddenly made the committee uncomfortable. Perhaps it was concerned that presenting the scene in public would be somehow seen as endorsing doctor-assisted suicide. While the committee agreed that the topic was an important one that needed to be discussed and explored, it was worried about forcing tourists and bystanders on Main Street to unwittingly engage in an interactive performance about death and dying.

Presenting the scene in a medical setting, within the framework of medical education, was one thing, but performing it for citizens in a public forum was quite another. Judging from the tone of the woman's voice, the hospital seemed on the verge of canceling the event altogether. She wanted to know if my company would be willing to go forward without *Women of Trachis*. She suggested that we find either another, less exposed venue or simply omit the scene altogether.

Though I was a bit taken aback, the request did not seem to warrant canceling the performance. I assured the public relations rep that we would be willing to follow the committee's recommendation and present only scenes from Sophocles's *Philoctetes*. But I also warned her that the questions I would ask during the audience discussion would remain unchanged. As facilitator, I would pull no punches. The conversation would be no different than if we had performed *Women of Trachis*, and if I didn't believe we could achieve the same level of openness and candor with scenes from *Philoctetes*, I wouldn't entertain the idea of proceeding with the performance.

At the time, I thought little of the call. We had received requests from communities before, asking us to modify aspects of performances to meet the needs of specific audiences. Though no one had asked us to omit a scene before, I saw this instance as no different from ones in which we had altered an event's marketing or reframed the facilitator's questions to best engage a target audience. Besides, the project's objective wasn't to make a political point. Ever since I'd cared for Laura, I'd had one message to deliver—that our society should be devoting as much time, resources, and discussion to end-of-life care as, for the last twenty-five years, we have dedicated to childbirth. Also, offending or enraging the hospital executives who were bringing the project to Falmouth would serve absolutely no one. We made the requested change in the program, updated the flyer, and moved on.

Little did we know that the hospital's decision to omit *Women of Trachis* would bring far more attention to Sophocles's least-known play than had we performed it at top volume on the town square.

About a week later, an article entitled "Hospital Nixes Portion of Reading from Classic Greek Play" ran in the *Cape Cod Times*. Then a series of letters to the editor ran in a local biweekly, the *Falmouth Enterprise*:

UPSET WITH ETHICS COMMITTEE

Businesses up and down Main Street must be on their knees giving thanks to Falmouth Hospital's decision to censor Tuesday night's Sophocles show on the library lawn.

Artie's: Put in more clams. Roo Bar: Get those daiquiri blenders a' whirring. Tuesday's shaping up to be a big midweek payday.

Because we, who just heard that Sophocles might be too deep or too dirty, are about to come runnin.'

Thank you, hospital ethics committee—you, the very same "First, do no harm" blokes, after all. Thank you for your learned decision to prevent a "passerby from being piqued."

If you pique a passerby, will he not bleed out? Or will he not cry "Lawsuit! I'm too stupid and/ or my sensibilities too delicate for your 5th century Greek theater"?

Has anybody taken a good look at the average passerby lately? The ethics committee has got no worries about piquing this fellow. He's so bored, so tuned out, he strides down the street not looking up or down or sideways, but into the palm of his hand at his iPad, iPhone, iWhatever. He cries out to be offended, to be piqued, to be whatever you keep him from being.

Falmouth is a lot of things, but a cultural backwater it is not. The ethics committee deserves all the shame, ridicule, and piquing it gets for offending this passerby in the crudest way possible: with its boorish condescension.

Anne L. Macaulay
Meadow Lane
Falmouth

CENSORING THE CENSOR

It is unfortunate that some educated and respected members of our community have reached a conclusion without investigating the facts. At no time have I ever, either publicly or confidentially, recommended that the dramatic readings by Sophocles be censored, abridged, or in any way "banned." This is a gross misstatement of my suggestion (not edict!) that a venue be found wherein interested listeners would have the opportunity to decide if this production was one they chose to hear.

Autonomy applies to free speech as much as to healthcare decisions, and exposing casual passersby on a summer evening to this intense drama would be in effect acting without their informed consent. It is time for us all to address the serious ethical issues pertaining to decision-making at the end of life in an appropriate forum.

Jane Schweitzer, M.D.
Chairman
Upper Cape Ethics Committee

WATCHING NOT MANDATORY
Had I known sooner that grand-motherhood would include being protected by well-meaning people from the likes of Sophocles, I might not have signed up for the gig.

Disinterested or offended passersby could just choose to speed up their passing by.

Anne M. Corwin
Shore Street
Falmouth

Whether or not it amounted to censorship, the ethics committee's action had clearly touched a nerve in Falmouth. And in the days leading up to the performance, aggrieved residents continued to voice their indignation and concern at what they perceived to be blatant paternalism on the part of the hospital. The tireless spirit and independence of thought long associated with the self-determined residents of New England remained on full display, as a number of them sent us unsolicited e-mails professing solidarity and promising protests on behalf of Sophocles's play. A local librarian wrote to ask for permission to use my translation. She was planning a public reading of *Women of Trachis* in September, for Banned Books Week, and was also designing a display for the library lobby, featuring, among other banned titles, Sophocles's play.

Never had more discussion been generated in anticipation of one of our performances than that summer in Falmouth, and when we finally arrived on July 19, the town was bristling with outrage and a collective desire to talk about it. By six-thirty p.m., the neatly manicured lawn in front of the library began to fill with octogenarians, ambling slowly and deliberately across the grass to plant themselves on lawn chairs near the loudspeakers on either side of the stage. By seven, close to two hundred people, most of them appearing to be over seventy, had come of their own volition to discuss death on the public square.

One of the main reasons I had agreed to follow the ethics committee's recommendation is that Sophocles's *Philoctetes* contains a scene that is strikingly similar to the controversial one in *Women of Trachis*. Philoctetes asks a young man named Neoptolemus—in no uncertain terms—to help him end his life. As in *Women of Trachis*, the request is made in the middle of a gruesome attack, as Philoctetes's body is ravaged by a cruel disease. The difference is that Philoctetes suffers from a chronic condition, while Heracles's affliction is terminal. Between screams, the suffering warrior attempts to persuade the young man, roughly the same age as Heracles's son Hyllus, to "release him" from the grip of pain, even referring in his plea to Heracles's famous death by immolation. In one variant of the Heracles myth, it was Philoctetes who lit the fire and burned Heracles alive, for which Heracles gave him his invincible bow.

PHILOCTETES
DEATH! DEATH! DEATH!
Where are you? Why, after
all these years of calling,
have you not appeared?
My noble son, take my body,
scorch it on a raging fire,
as I once burned the owner
of the bow that you now hold.

Why the silence?
Say something.
Where have you gone?

NEOPTOLEMUS
Your pain is painful to observe.

PHILOCTETES
It comes as quickly as it goes.
Be brave. I beg you to stay.

NEOPTOLEMUS
Don't worry. We will stay.

PHILOCTETES
You will?

NEOPTOLEMUS
Without a doubt!

As the actor Jeff Zinn moaned and wailed in agony, belting Philoctetes's cries so loudly across the square that they ricocheted off surrounding buildings and came bouncing back on all sides like a chorus of screams, the gray- and blue-haired members of the audience leaned forward in their lawn chairs and took in the performance with rapt attention. It was as if at some point in their lives, they had all screamed this way, if not aloud, then in their minds. By performing Philoctetes's existential agony, Zinn was screaming on their behalf.

On the other side of the square, a group of teenagers milled down Main Street past ice cream parlors, bars, and restaurants, listening to the performance and exhibiting a completely different response. Every time Philoctetes screamed, they—mockingly—screamed back, matching his intensity and volume but with an equal measure of derision. This back-and-forth continued for most of the scene. But the audience didn't seem to hear the chorus of young voices on the periphery poking fun at the earnest exercise in front of the library.

As I observed both groups, I found myself grinning from ear to ear. Of course, the aged audience would treat suffering and death with reverence and humility. They were running out of time. And of course the adolescents would arrogantly laugh in the face of death. In their own minds, they were immortal. But the people who showed up that night to hear and discuss Sophocles's ancient play had come with a singular purpose. If they didn't come together as a community to talk about death that summer night, when would they?

After the performance ended and the actors took seats in the audience, a few people—at first—expressed anger about the exclusion of *Women of Trachis* from the program. But once that sentiment had been properly voiced, the conversation quickly turned to the matter at hand. A registered nurse stood up and talked about how distressing it was when a professional caregiver, such as a home health aide, cares for a patient for months or years, then is pushed to the sidelines by a family member who arrives from out of town at the last minute, right before the patient dies. Another man recounted the death of his father, relating it to the suffering of Philoctetes. "His pain was painful to observe," he said, quoting Neoptolemus.

One woman described how a close friend who was dying had refused painkillers and other drugs because he wanted to be fully present for death, which he believed was the last thing he would experience in life. The chief of palliative care at the hospital talked about the power of morphine and other opiates to alleviate suffering and ease patients toward death.

I took a moment to talk about the "double effect,"

a legal protocol employed in most medical settings to mitigate suffering and facilitate the dying process. Suppose someone complains of physical pain, and a nurse or a doctor administers medication to treat it. If the secondary effect of the drugs is the suppression of the respiratory system and, ultimately, death, that's okay, because the primary intent was to relieve suffering. From my experience caring for Laura and spending time with hospice and palliative care nurses, the so-called double effect seemed to be the eight-hundred-pound gorilla of end-of-life care—the biggest, most-closeted secret in the profession, a legally sanctioned way to help people who are suffering to die. However, it is also one of the least understood, and perhaps most destructive, concepts in end-of-life care, which often leads caregivers and family members to feel that they are somehow responsible for terminally ill patients' deaths.

As the sun descended onto the horizon and the final rays of summer light faded, a cool evening breeze moved over the crowd. A doctor signaled to me, asking for the microphone. He stood up, composed himself, and like a chorus leader, addressed the audience: "We cannot prevent death. Life will end. Most doctors, I'm ashamed to say, spend most of their time prolonging illness. Life is a terminal condition. No one walks away from it." Heads silently nodded in agreement, and for a brief moment, nothing more needed to be said.

As the audience slowly filed out across the Falmouth town square, lawn chairs in tow, it dawned on me, perhaps for the first time, that all my work with Greek tragedy since Laura's death had been in service of one thing: surrounding myself with people who wanted to face the darkness together and tell their stories. Perhaps that's what—above all—ancient Greek tragedy was designed to do. I often get asked, "Where is the hope in all these tragedies you perform?" The hope is not in the plays but in the people who come together to bear witness to their truth. If these ancient tragedies can teach us anything today, it's how to listen to one another without judgment, how to grow from our experiences and mistakes, and how to heal as one community. That, I've learned, is where hope can be found in tragedy.

EPILOGUE

In the early days of Theater of War, I followed a hunch about ancient Greek tragedies that led us to unexpected audiences in unlikely places, and gave me a new understanding of the relationship between theater and audience. But these days Outside the Wire sometimes seems more like the fire department than a theater company. A call comes in, we design a new project, and then we deploy our actors to the community in need.

The first call came in 2011, after an EF5 tornado roughly three-quarters of a mile wide—one of the largest in recorded history—flattened a large swath of the city of Joplin, Missouri, killing 161 people and destroying more than 7,000 apartments and homes in 32 minutes. George Lombardi, the state's director of corrections who had hosted our first performances of Prometheus in Prison, traveled to Joplin to survey the damage. When he saw the indescribable wreckage—piles of cars stacked up like children's blocks, churches and nursing homes torn from their foundations, and fields of splintered debris where homes, schools, and hospitals had once stood—he wrote to me and asked,

"Is there a story that might help the people of Joplin begin to come to terms with what has happened here?"

I replied with a single suggestion, the *Book of Job,* an ancient Hebrew poem about a righteous, prosperous man who is tested by God when he loses everything—his children, his crops, his livestock, his house, and his health—after a great wind annihilates his home. Convinced of his own innocence, Job sits silently in the dirt behind what's left of his home and asks God for an explanation. But God doesn't answer.

A group of friends visit Job. At first they sympathize with his suffering, but when he questions why he has been singled out and made to suffer, they condemn him and say he must have done something to deserve his terrible fate. But Job clings to the belief that he has done nothing wrong and continues to shake his fists at the sky in righteous indignation.

At the very end of the poem, God reveals Himself to Job in a disembodied voice from within a whirlwind and rebukes him for presuming to understand His will. Job covers his mouth and falls silent, and—in an enigmatic ending—God restores his health and prosperity, doubling his children, his livestock, and his crops.

For thousands of years, people have sought comfort in this story and its timeless exploration of how humans behave when disaster strikes.

We premiered the Book of Job project in Joplin, Missouri, for more than a thousand people in a Christian megachurch, then later, on the eve of the one-year anniversary of the tornado, we performed it in a high school auditorium. We used Stephen Mitchell's beautiful, dramatically charged translation. The actor Paul Giamatti played Job, David Strathairn played God, and Arliss Howard played the Narrator. When the survivors of the Joplin tornado saw and heard their own experiences reflected in the performance of an ancient biblical poem, they opened up and shared their stories and perspectives. They grappled with what it meant, one year later, to move forward with their lives, while still living with reverence and respect for those who were lost. Here is how people in Joplin responded to the Book of Job performances:

"No matter what, when a person openly, honestly, truthfully pours out their heart and soul, I must listen openly, honestly, without judgment or prejudice."

"I'm a survivor. The midwesterner in me, the Joplin boy in me, wants to hear the last word be . . . okay. We got hurt, we grieved, shook our fists at the heavens, cleaned up, went to work. . . . Let's move on."

"If you tell people they need to move on, maybe it's you who needs them to move on."

"Though I lost my home to a tornado in 2011 and to a tree in 2007 and almost lost my life to six natural events in the last six years, I didn't think

I could relate to Job until Paul [Giamatti] spoke his words!"

"I talked to a lady after the tornado—she said she wished she had died instead of a friend. I think she was in so much pain. I listened, but I wish I could have known what to say. She had lost hope. She definitely was wanting to curse God. All I could do was pray and I cried. I now wish I had said nothing and just held her. Words aren't always helpful."

"The text reminds us of our common humanity across time and generations."

"It was comforting to see that we are all human."

"Suffering transcends time."

I have heard variations of this final comment in almost every community we have visited, regardless of the prevailing language, culture, or religion. And what I have seen in the faces of audience members—night after night—is a palpable sense of relief to discover that they are not the only people in the world to have felt such feelings. I would go so far as to suggest that audience members are, in a way, healed by the realization that they are not alone in their communities, not alone in the world, and not alone across time. Or as one Vietnam veteran named Jay F. Johnson eloquently put it after an early performance of Theater of War at the Juilliard School of Drama in New York City, "Knowing that PTSD goes back to BC gives me the feeling I'm not totally alone."

What I've learned from this work is that if you want to have a discussion about a subject that divides us or makes us uncomfortable, always begin with a portrayal of human suffering. Through empathy, imagination, and shared discomfort, we often find a common language as well as common ground. Tragedy, both theatrical and personal, knows no boundaries. No one can be protected from it. Ancient tragedies, in particular, hold the power to dissolve and transcend all the artificial walls that we humans work so hard to build around ourselves.

Months after Hurricane Sandy tore a wide path of destruction through New York City, Marjorie Slome, the rabbi of West End Temple in Rockaway, Queens, contacted me. Rockaway was perhaps one of the hardest-hit areas—the water had surged dangerously high on both sides of the narrow spit of peninsula at the base of Long Island where the synagogue sat, flooding its halls with more than five feet of water. She had heard about our performances of the Book of Job in Joplin after the tornado and wondered if we might perform Job for her congregation on the anniversary of Sandy, in the ruins of the main sanctuary.

I agreed, and as word of the synagogue performance spread throughout the city, we were also invited to perform in a number of other places that the storm had leveled: a community theater at a decommissioned military base, an African American church, a senior center, an elementary school in an impoverished neighborhood, and a fire station, to name a few. Wherever we performed, no matter who was in the audience, the responses were remarkably similar to those we first encountered in Joplin.

One of the most memorable performances took place in the recently rebuilt sanctuary of a church in Far Rockaway. First Sandy had washed it out; then months later a reckless driver had lost control, careened off the street, and rammed his SUV into the building, straight through a brick wall. The church had nearly burned to the ground. Needless to say, no one in the audience that night was unfamiliar with Job's despair. After the reading, a man addressed the audience, gripping the microphone with trembling hands, and took the risk of sharing his story, a timeless one that seemed to capture the essence of the raw feelings vibrating through the room.

He had served in the NYPD in various capacities for more than twenty years. During that time, he had been shot at, threatened, and exposed to violence. He had risked his life countless times in service of the greater good, with a core belief that actions matter in the world, that the world is held together by something akin to karma, some semblance of moral causality. After

9/11, he had been sent to the Middle East to gather intelligence on terrorist groups plotting future attacks on New York City. He had pursued and helped capture those who would take the lives of innocent civilians, averting unimaginable bloodshed here at home. Like Job, he considered himself a righteous, God-fearing person, who had struggled his entire life to do the right thing, even at great personal cost. So it came as quite a shock when, a few weeks after relocating his family to a beautiful new home in Rockaway, Queens, directly next to the ocean, the skies had opened up, the seas had swelled, and though no one was hurt, everything he had worked for and built had been destroyed in an instant.

The next morning the rain finally stopped, the ocean receded, and the sun peeked through clouds illuminating the pile of rubble that had once been his dream home. He stood in his front yard, speechlessly surveying the damage. A neighbor walked up and stood by his side. "Is there anything you need?" he quietly asked.

The man paused, unable to formulate his thoughts, let alone the words that could convey the tempest of emotions churning through him. "I guess . . . I guess I could use a shovel," he replied.

The neighbor brought him one and left him there alone, standing in the debris, to begin digging. The man gripped the shovel tightly, then raised his fist at the sky, and with tears streaming down his face, he repeated the words that Job once cried out to his maker: "You have *not* treated me justly!"

Heads moved in the Rockaway church pews with

tacit understanding, while a few audience members vocalized sounds of shared grief, loss, and commiseration, like a Greek chorus singing softly, and in unison, at the foot of the altar.

Over the past few years, Outside the Wire has continued to expand the work that started with Theater of War. We've presented Euripides's *Bacchae* in drug-ravaged towns in Appalachia, and Seneca's *Thyestes* for survivors of political violence and torture. We've performed modern classics inspired by Greek tragedies, such as Eugene O'Neill's *A Long Day's Journey into Night* for primary care physicians and recovering addicts, and Tennessee Williams's *A Streetcar Named Desire* for rural communities in Maine affected by an epidemic of domestic violence.

And we've presented contemporary plays by writers such as Conor McPherson and Stephen Belber on U.S. Army bases in Japan, Kuwait, and Qatar, to help address issues such as alcohol abuse and sexual assault in the military. Not all the texts we perform these days are tragedies, in the strict sense of the word, but all depict powerful, universal human experiences through elevated poetic language and dramatic action. And all the plays we choose, even the contemporary ones, are distant enough from the audiences for whom we perform, by way of culture or time, to create a safe space for open dialogue.

In 2014, through a partnership with the Global

Mental Health Program at Columbia University, we embarked on our first international project: we presented dramatic readings of a fifteenth-century Noh play called *Sumidagawa*, about a grieving mother, for survivors of the 3/11 earthquake, tsunami, and nuclear disaster in Japan. The first reading of the play, in Japanese, was for a group of mothers who had relocated their children from Fukushima to Tokyo after the disaster.

Given how profoundly reluctant the Japanese are—as a culture—to share their emotions, our partners in Japan were worried that no one would dare to speak during the audience discussion. But soon after the actors had finished the reading, the mothers began to open up and share their stories, using the language of the play as a bridge to their own experiences. In fact, one of the biggest complaints we received that day was that we had allotted only an hour for the discussion. Listening, through a translator, to the mothers speak about surviving the disaster and then, over several years, attempting to rebuild their lives, all the while struggling to maintain a sense of normalcy, safety, and security for their children, I was overwhelmed with emotions. In the end, the Japanese audience seemed no different from any other audience that we had performed for in the past. Now that we have established that our work can reach even the most reticent of cultures, the possibilities for future projects seem limitless.

ACKNOWLEDGMENTS

Since founding Theater of War, I have enjoyed the true privilege of hearing people of all walks of life—all over the world—tell candid, courageous stories that have reaffirmed my faith in humans and our ability to survive, adapt, and change. I have met individuals whose inner strength in the face of unimaginable trauma and loss has taught me never to underestimate anyone. Because of these audience members, on account of their insights and bravery, I have found a way to merge my love of classics, translation, and performance into a public service. It is from them that I have learned the purpose of tragedy, and for that I will forever be grateful. I lack the words to convey my appreciation for them all, but I would like to express my sincere thanks to Jeff and Sheri Hall, George Adkinson, and Leslie Blackhall for generously allowing me to interview them for this book and for permitting me to share their stories with an even larger audience.

There are many other individuals whose friendship, feedback, collaboration, and support have made this manuscript possible. I would like to thank my agent,

Zoë Pagnamenta, for believing in this book and for convincing me to write it. I would like to thank my editor, Andrew Miller, for his steady-handed guidance and patience over these past few years and for trusting me to write this book. And I would like to offer my special thanks and deepest gratitude to the following interlocutors and readers for poring over this text at various stages in its development and for providing invaluable comments and criticism: Sally Arteseros, Sarah Botstein, Noam Elcott, Sarah Levitt, Wyatt Mason, Bill Mullen, Jim Ottaway, and Geoffrey C. Ward. Heartfelt thanks also go to my producing partner, Phyllis Kaufman, for her expansive vision and tireless dedication to Outside the Wire and our many projects. I would also like to thank the scores of gifted actors who, through limitless passion and artistry, have made our projects come to life. Readers can find a list of their names on our website, but it seems fitting to mention a few who were with us when we got started and are still with us today: Bill Camp, Reg E. Cathey, Keith David, Adam Driver, Jesse Eisenberg, Giancarlo Esposito, Zach Grenier, Paul Giamatti, Bill Irwin, Brían F. O'Byrne, Elizabeth Marvel, Jay O. Sanders, David Strathairn, Michael Stuhlbarg, Lili Taylor, and Joanne Tucker.

Over the years, many mentors have made a difference in my life, but I feel compelled to mention a few, whose generosity toward me and influence upon my work cannot be measured. They are my late father Lee Doerries, Marielle Bancou-Segal, Leon Botstein, Michael Brint, Peter Brook, Cliff Faulkner, Margo Figgins, Keith

Fowler, Connie Holmes, Eugen Kullmann, Harvey Lichtenstein, Bill McCulloh, David Rath, Robert Weimann, and Andrew Zolli. I also want to acknowledge Marcia Childress, Chuck Engel, Mary Hull, Lyuba Konopasek, George Lombardi, Bill Nash, and Loree Sutton, all early adopters, whose willingness to take risks on behalf of the projects helped blaze a path for them. My thanks also go to Ken Burns, Joe DePlasco, Marie-Hélène Estienne, the Hunter Gohl family, Taylor Krauss, Lynn Novick, Drew Patrick, Ransom Riggs, Jamie Romm, Mary Rothenberg, Jonathan Shay, Andrew Solomon, Felicitas Thorne, and Elisabeth Turnauer for their friendship and belief in my work. I also wish to thank my mother, Denyse Doerries, and my brother, Mark Doerries, as well as my extended family for their love and support.

Finally, I would like to thank my amazing daughter, Abigail, for inspiring me each day to be a better person and for filling my life with laughter and light. And most significantly, I wish to thank my wife, Sarah, who is the strongest person I know, for guiding me back to the world of the living, supporting my vision from the beginning, and pushing me to pursue my dreams—no matter how impractical—wherever they should lead. Without her enduring love, unwavering faith, boundless energy, and extraordinary courage, none of this would have ever happened.

NOTES

PROLOGUE

4 **According to a 2012 Veterans Affairs study**: Janet Kemp and Robert Bossarte, "Suicide Data Report, 2012," *Department of Veterans Affairs* (February 2012): 15.

LEARNING THROUGH SUFFERING

11 **Ironically, some scholars now suggest**: Winkler, "Ephebes' Song," 31.

12 **Also, as Aristotle pointed out**: Aristotle, *Poetics,* trans. Halliwell, 44.

16 **But as many as 60 percent of type 2 diabetics**: David F. Blackburn, Jaris Swidrovich, and Mark Lemstra, "Non-adherence in Type-2 diabetes: Practical Considerations for Interpreting the Literature," *Journal of Patient Preference and Adherence* 7 (March 2013): 183–89.

18 **Hispanic Americans are at a "particularly high risk for type 2 diabetes"**: "Check Your Risk for Developing Type 2 Diabetes," Centers for Disease Control and Prevention (March 26, 2012).

21 **"A young man cannot have"**: Nietzsche, *We Philologists,* 110.

21 **"The philologist," he writes**: Ibid., 113.

21 **"Old men are well suited"**: Ibid.

22 **"In short," he concludes**: Ibid., 110.

23 **"representation of an action"**: Aristotle, *Poetics,* trans. Halliwell, 37.

23 **"Tragedy," he writes**: Ibid.

23 **"A person's character is his fate"**: Heraclitus, *Fragments,* trans. Robinson, Fragment 119, p. 69.

27 **"an object or an act becomes real"**: Eliade, *Myth of Eternal Return,* 34.

35 **The goal of eliciting these emotions**: Aristotle, *Poetics,* trans. Halliwell, 37.

36 **"all poetical imitations are ruinous"**: Plato, *Republic,* trans. Jowett, Book 10.

37 **In 1993 a team of psychologists**: B. S. McEwen and E. Stellar, "Stress and the Individual: Mechanisms Leading to Disease," *Archives of Internal Medicine* 18 (September 1993): 2093–2101.

43 **"as if they were well-informed and matured men"**: Nietzsche, *We Philologists,* 147.

PTSD IS FROM BC

61 **"Behind the door of Army Spec."**: Priest and Hull, "Soldiers Face Neglect."

63 **"Imagine my surprise"**: Doerries, trans., *All That You've Seen Here Is God,* 147.

64 **Roughly 95 percent of the injured**: Alan Cullison, "On Distant Battle Fields, Survival Odds Rise Sharply," *Wall Street Journal,* April 2, 2010.

64 **more than thirty thousand veterans**: "DoD Worldwide Numbers for TBI," Defense and Veterans Brain Injury Center, 2014.

67 **"Town by town across the country"**: Sontag and Alvarez, "Across America, Deadly Echoes of Foreign Battles."

68 **"What should I do now?"**: Doerries, trans., *All That You've Seen Here Is God*, 46.

75 **Dr. Jonathan Shay**: Shay, "Birth of Tragedy."

77 **"We must create our own"**: Shay, *Achilles in Vietnam*, 94.

77 **The archeological record suggests**: Winkler, "Ephebes' Song," 38.

79 **"How can I say"**: Doerries, trans., *All That You've Seen Here Is God*, 29.

80 **"I call upon the Furies"**: Ibid., 74.

82 **"Ahhhhhhhhhhhhhhhhhh!"**: Ibid., 171.

88 **"You are either going to help me"**: Murphy, "Soldier Faces 5 Murder Charges."

89 **It was then that she noticed him losing sleep**: "Accused GI's Mental Health Debated in Iraq Shootings," Associated Press, August 10, 2011.

89 **"made him feel like he wanted to kill somebody"**: Murphy, "Soldier Faces 5 Murder Charges."

90 **"I experienced it as being aggressive and hostile,"**: Ibid.

90 **According to his defense attorney**: Murphy, "Did the System Fail a Soldier?"

91 **Soldiers from his unit observed him weeping**: "Army Sergeant Pleads Guilty to Killing 5 in Baghdad," Associated Press, April 26, 2013.

91 **Any service member who "strikes his superior"**: Article 90, *Uniform Code of Military Justice*.

92 **"to say an arrogant word"**: Doerries, trans., *All That You've Seen Here Is God*, 23.

93 **"I feel sorry for him"**: Ibid., 22.

94 **"though he had not been struck"**: Herodotus, *The Landmark Herodotus: The Histories*, trans. Purvis, 6.117, p. 490.

94 **And in perhaps the most gruesome**: For a compelling exploration of this argument, see Meagher, *Heracles Gone Mad: Rethinking Heroism in an Age of Endless War.*

95 **"children fainted and unborn infants were aborted"**: Quoted in Lefkowitz, *Lives of Greek Poets,* 74.

97 **Startlingly, a study**: M. Friedman, "Suicide Risk Among Soldiers: Early Findings from Army Study to Assess Risk and Resilience in Servicemembers," *JAMA Psychiatry* 71 (May 2014): 487–89.

98 **"I call out to Hermes"**: Doerries, trans., *All That You've Seen Here Is God,* 74.

101 **During the American Civil War**: Steve Bentley, "A Short History of PTSD: From Thermopylae to Hue, Soldiers Have Always Had a Disturbing Reaction to War," *VVA Veteran* 1 (1991): 1.

101 **In 1905 the Russian army coined**: Gabriel, *No More Heroes,* 109.

103 **"the persistence into civilian life"**: Quoted in Schmidle, "In the Crosshairs," 34.

103 **"betrayal of 'what's right'"**: Shay, *Achilles in Vietnam,* 5.

107 **"Ajax./Ajax./My name is a sad song"**: Doerries, trans., *All That You've Seen Here Is God,* 44.

AMERICAN AJAX

111 **Ajax could no longer remember**: In this section, and others like it throughout the book, I attempt to imagine and frame the circumstances leading up to the dramatic events depicted by the ancient plays. These meditations on the thoughts and experiences of characters like Ajax have been generated in much the same manner that actors and directors develop and shape the inner lives of characters, i.e., through imagination and play. They

are not meant to serve as historical or even mythological records, but rather as improvisations upon the plays designed to bring the reader closer to the motivations and struggles at the heart of each tragedy.

133 **"Think about your father"**: Doerries, trans., *All That You've Seen Here Is God*, 49.

152 **"Oh Ajax, this was no way"**: Ibid., 81.

PROMETHEUS IN SOLITARY

156 **"6.98 million offenders"**: Lauren E. Glaze and Erica Parks, "Correctional Populations in the United States, 2011," Bureau of Justice Statistics, November 2012.

157 **And of those, roughly 25,000**: Gawande, "Hellhole," 42.

160 **The average direct cost, per prisoner**: "Missouri Reentry Process," Missouri Department of Corrections, 2012.

168 **"Why have you come?"**: Doerries, trans., *All That You've Seen Here Is God*, 257.

171 **"I saved men"**: Ibid., 250.

174 **The prisoners were released on bail**: Pickard-Cambridge, *Dramatic Festivals of Athens*, 59.

175 **According to fifth-century-BC Athenian law**: Plato, *Laws*, 9:865–66.

176 **"Solitude is the primary condition"**: Foucault, *Discipline and Punish*, 237.

176 **"One of the paradoxes of solitary"**: Gawande, "Hellhole," 40.

177 **at least 95 percent of all prisoners**: Timothy Hughes and Doris James Wilson, "Reentry Trends in the U.S.," Bureau of Justice Statistics, 2014.

179 **"So let the lightning"**: Doerries, trans., *All That You've Seen Here Is God*, 336.

197 **"Witness / how the gods"**: Ibid., 236.

199 **The strike ended**: "New Hunger Strike Begins After the

Department of Defense Reneges on Promises to Detainees," Center for Constitutional Rights, August 31, 2005.

200 **"both detainee lawyers and military officials"**: Savage, "Guantánamo Hunger Strike Largely Over."

201 **"Prometheus. / I groan"**: Doerries, trans., *All That You've Seen Here Is God*, 230.

205 **"Boldly spoken"**: Ibid., 326.

208 **"Oh Mother!"**: Ibid., 340.

HERACLES IN HOSPICE

215 **"It has me in its teeth"**: Doerries, trans., *All That You've Seen Here Is God*, 430.

216 **"Father, what / are you saying?"**: Ibid., 454.

218 **cults worshipping Asclepius**: Wickkiser, *Asklepios, Medicine, and Politics of Healing*, 78.

219 **"Given the Greek belief"**: Mitchell-Boyask, "Plague and Theater in Ancient Athens," 374–75.

220 **"language is the healer of the soul"**: August Meineke, comp., *Fragmenta Comicorum Graecorum* (Berolini: Typis et Empensis G. Reimeri, 1841), 4:240.

221 **"A savage pestilence"**: Sophocles, *Oedipus the King*, trans. Bryan Doerries, unpublished.

225 **"do away with the sufferings"**: Hippocrates of Cos, *Art*, 193.

227 **"It seems this boy"**: Doerries, trans., *All That You've Seen Here Is God*, 458.

229 **"Then you order"**: Ibid., 459.

231 **the ethical insight of Greek tragedy resides**: Hunter, "Limiting Treatment in a Social Vacuum," 716.

231 **"presence and its sympathy"**: Ibid.

233 **"Hoist him upon your"**: Doerries, trans., *All That You've Seen Here Is God*, 462.

250 **About a week later, an article**: Sean Teehan, "Hospital

Nixes Portion of Reading from Classic Greek Play," *Cape Cod Times,* July 15, 2011.

250 **"Upset with Ethics Committee"**: "Letters to the Editor," *Falmouth Enterprise,* July 15, 2011, 4–5.

254 **"DEATH! DEATH! DEATH!"**: Doerries, trans., *All That You've Seen Here Is God,* 171.

BIBLIOGRAPHY

Aristotle. *Poetics of Aristotle.* Translated by Steven Halliwell. Chapel Hill: University of North Carolina Press, 1987.

Boal, Augusto. *Theatre of the Oppressed.* Translated by Charles A. McBride. New York: Theatre Communications Group, 1993.

Brook, Peter. *The Empty Space: A Book About the Theatre: Deadly, Holy, Rough, Immediate.* Reprint ed. New York: Touchstone, 1995.

————. *The Shifting Point: Theater, Film, Opera 1946–1987.* New York: Theatre Communications Group, 1994.

Campbell, Joseph. *The Hero with a Thousand Faces.* 3rd ed. Novato, Calif.: New World Library, 2008.

————. *The Power of Myth.* New York: Anchor Books, 1991.

Dodds, E. R. *The Greeks and the Irrational.* Berkeley: University of California Press, 1951.

Doerries, Bryan, trans. *All That You've Seen Here Is God: New Translations of Four Greek Tragedies.* New York: Vintage, 2015.

Easterling, P. E., ed. *The Cambridge Companion to Ancient Greek Tragedy.* Cambridge, U.K.: Cambridge University Press, 1997.

Eliade, Mircea. *The Myth of the Eternal Return: Cosmos and History.* Translated by Willard R. Trask. Princeton, N.J.: Princeton University Press, 2005.

Foucault, Michel. *Discipline and Punish: The Birth of the Prison.* Translated by Alan Sheridan. 2nd ed. New York: Vintage, 1995.

Gabriel, Richard A. *No More Heroes: Madness and Psychiatry in War.* New York: Hill and Wang, 1988.

Gawande, Atul. "Hellhole: The United States Holds Tens of Thousands of Inmates in Long-Term Solitary Confinement. Is This Torture?" *New Yorker,* March 30, 2009.

Graves, Robert. *The Greek Myths.* Combined ed. New York: Penguin, 1992.

Hedges, Chris. *War Is a Force That Gives Us Meaning.* New York: Anchor, 2002.

Heraclitus. *Fragments.* Translated by T. M. Robinson. Toronto: University of Toronto Press, 1987.

Herodotus. *The Landmark Herodotus: The Histories.* Translated by Adrea L. Purvis. Edited by Robert B. Strassler. New York: Anchor Books, 2009.

Hippocrates of Cos. *The Art.* Translated by W. H. S. Jones. Loeb Classical Library 148. Cambridge, Mass.: Harvard University Press, 1959.

Hunter, Kathryn M. "Limiting Treatment in a Social Vacuum." *Archives of Internal Medicine* 145 (April 1985): 716–19.

Kitto, H. D. F. *Greek Tragedy: A Literary Study.* London and New York: Routledge, 1939.

Knox, Bernard. *Oedipus at Thebes: Sophocles' Tragic Hero and His Time.* New Haven, Conn.: Yale University Press, 1957.

Lefkowitz, Mary R. *The Lives of the Greek Poets.* Baltimore: Johns Hopkins University Press, 1981.

Marlantes, Karl. *What It Is Like to Go to War.* New York: Atlantic Monthly Press, 2010.

Mason, Wyatt. "You Are Not Alone Across Time: Using Sophocles to Treat PTSD." *Harper's Magazine,* October 2014.

Meagher, Robert Emmet. *Heracles Gone Mad: Rethinking Heroism in an Age of Endless War.* Northampton, Mass.: Olive Branch Press, 2006.

Mitchell-Boyask, Robin. *Plague and the Athenian Imagination: Drama, History, and the Cult of Asclepios.* Cambridge, U.K.: Cambridge University Press, 2011.

———. "Plague and Theater in Ancient Athens." *Lancet* 373 (January 31, 2009): 374–75.

Murphy, Kim. "Did the System Fail a Soldier?" *Los Angeles Times,* April 15, 2013.

———. "Soldier Faces 5 Murder Charges in 2009 Shootings at Iraq Clinic." *Los Angeles Times,* May 18, 2012.

Nietzsche, Friedrich. *The Birth of Tragedy and Other Writings.* Translated by Ronald Speirs. Edited by Raymond Guess and Ronald Speirs. Cambridge, U.K.: Cambridge University Press, 1999.

———. *We Philologists.* Translated by J. M. Kennedy. Edinburgh: T. N. Foulis, 1911.

Palaima, Thomas G. "Civilian Knowledge of War and Violence in Ancient Athens and Modern America." In *Experiencing War: Trauma and Society from Ancient Greece to the Iraq War.* Edited by Michael B. Cosmopoulos. Chicago: Ares Publishers, 2007.

Pickard-Cambridge, Sir Arthur. *The Dramatic Festivals of Athens.* Edited by John Gould and D. M. Lewis. 2nd ed. Oxford, U.K.: Clarendon Press, 1968.

Plato. *The Republic.* Translated by Benjamin Jowett. Internet Classics Archive. Oxford, U.K.: Clarendon Press, 1894.

Priest, Dana, and Anne Hull. "Soldiers Face Neglect, Frustration at Army's Top Medical Hospital." *Washington Post,* February 18, 2007.

Savage, Charlie. "Guantánamo Hunger Strike Largely Over, U.S. Says." *New York Times,* September 23, 2013.

Schmidle, Nicholas. "In the Crosshairs." *New Yorker,* June 3, 2013.

Shay, Jonathan. *Achilles in Vietnam: Combat Trauma and the Undoing of Character.* New York: Scribner, 1994.

———. "The Birth of Tragedy out of the Needs of Democracy." *Didaskalia: The Journal for Ancient Performance* 2, no. 2 (April 1995).

———. *Odysseus in America: Combat Trauma and the Trials of Homecoming.* New York: Scribner, 2002.

Sontag, Deborah, and Lizette Alvarez. "Across America, Deadly Echoes of Foreign Battles." *New York Times,* January 13, 2008.

Taplin, Oliver. *Greek Tragedy in Action.* 2nd ed. London and New York: Routledge, 2002.

Tritle, Lawrence A. *From Melos to My Lai: A Study in Survival.* London and New York: Routledge, 2000.

Wickkiser, Bronwen. *Asklepios, Medicine, and the Politics of Healing in Fifth-Century Greece: Between Cult and Craft.* Baltimore: Johns Hopkins University Press, 2008.

Winkler, John J. "The Ephebes' Song." In *Nothing to Do with Dionysus? Athenian Drama in Its Social Context.* Edited by John J. Winkler and Froma Zeitlin. Princeton, N.J.: Princeton University Press, 1992.

Winnington-Ingram, R. P. *Sophocles: An Interpretation.* Cambridge, U.K.: Cambridge University Press, 1980.